**W9-BZA-545**

# Praise for Peter Canning's previous book, *Paramedic*

"[An] absorbing chronicle of [Canning's] first year on the job . . . he succeeds in finding heroism in an important job done well."
—*Publishers Weekly*

"Both a personal story and a vivid portrait of his profession, one that despite its importance is often taken for granted . . . *Paramedic* deepened my appreciation for the work paramedics do."
—*The Washington Post*

"Fast-paced . . . Vivid . . . Eye-opening."
—*The Hartford Courant*

"A vivid account of emergency medicine that should go a long way toward generating respect for paramedics . . . [Canning's] daily life centers on the nitty-gritty of emergency medicine. . . . An unpredictable mix of tension, action, frustration."
—*Kirkus Reviews*

*Please turn the page for more reviews. . . .*

"A splendid work . . . Filled with scintillating yet astute vignettes of life and death . . . Canning not only captures the magic of working with patients in all sorts of acute medical and traumatic events but does so with considerable eloquence."
—RICHARD L. JUDD
President, Central Connecticut State University
Professor of Emergency Medical Sciences

"The book is not just a series of adventures. Canning shares his doubts as he looks back on the calls that didn't go exactly right. He reveals his impatience and his frustrations on the job. He relates his experience on the streets with the policies being set in the state office buildings on high. The poverty of people in the inner city, particularly the circumstances of the children, tear at his heart as he briefly touches their lives in an emergency."
—*Manchester Journal Inquirer* (CT)

By Peter Canning
*Published by The Random House Publishing Group:*

PARAMEDIC: On the Front Lines of Medicine
RESCUE 471: A Paramedic's Stories

# RESCUE 471

## A Paramedic's Stories

## Peter Canning

THE RANDOM HOUSE PUBLISHING GROUP • NEW YORK

A Ballantine Book
Published by The Random House Publishing Group
Copyright © 2000 by Peter Canning

All rights reserved under International and Pan-American Copyright Conventions. Published in the United States by The Random House Publishing Group, a division of Random House, Inc., New York, and simultaneously in Canada by Random House of Canada Limited, Toronto.

Ballantine and colophon are registered trademarks of Random House, Inc.

www.ballantinebooks.com

Library of Congress Catalog Number: 00-190080

ISBN: 0-8041-1882-5

Manufactured in the United States of America

First Edition: April 2000

10  9  8  7

To my father

. . . and then the wounded knight, Sir Urre, set him up weakly, and prayed Sir Launcelot heartily, saying: Courteous knight, I require thee for God's sake heal my wounds, for methinketh ever sithen ye came here my wounds grieve me not. Ah, my fair lord, said Sir Launcelot, Jesu would that I might help you; I shame me sore that I should be thus rebuked, for never was I able in worthiness to do so high a thing. Then Sir Launcelot kneeled down by the wounded knight. . . . And then he held up his hands, and looked into the east, saying secretly unto himself: Thou blessed Father, Son, and Holy Ghost, I beseech thee of thy mercy, that my simple worship and honesty be saved, and thou blessed Trinity, thou mayest give power to heal this sick knight by thy great virtue and grace of thee, but, Good Lord, never of myself. And then Sir Launcelot prayed Sir Urre to let him see his head; and then devoutly kneeling he ransacked the three wounds, that they bled a little, and forthwith all the wounds fair healed, and seemed as they had been whole a seven year. And in likewise he searched his body of other three wounds, and they healed in likewise; and then the last of all he searched the which was in his hand, and anon it healed fair.

Then King Arthur and all the kings and knights kneeled down and gave thankings and lovings unto God and to His Blessed Mother. And ever Sir Launcelot wept as he had been a child that had been beaten.

—"The Healing of Sir Urre"
*Le Morte D'Arthur*
Sir Thomas Malory

# Contents

INTRODUCTION . . . . . . . . . . . . . . . . . . . . . . . . . . . . . xv

ARTHUR . . . . . . . . . . . . . . . . . . . . . . . . . . . . . . . . . . . 1
   Kools . . . . . . . . . . . . . . . . . . . . . . . . . . . . . . . . . . . . . 3
   Arthur . . . . . . . . . . . . . . . . . . . . . . . . . . . . . . . . . . . . . 6
   Rescue 471 . . . . . . . . . . . . . . . . . . . . . . . . . . . . . . . . 14
   Kids . . . . . . . . . . . . . . . . . . . . . . . . . . . . . . . . . . . . . . 23

SAVING LIVES . . . . . . . . . . . . . . . . . . . . . . . . . . . . . 27
   Perfect . . . . . . . . . . . . . . . . . . . . . . . . . . . . . . . . . . . . 29
   No Luck Left . . . . . . . . . . . . . . . . . . . . . . . . . . . . . . 37
   Saving Lives . . . . . . . . . . . . . . . . . . . . . . . . . . . . . . 39
   Bag and Drag . . . . . . . . . . . . . . . . . . . . . . . . . . . . . 41
   Baby Code . . . . . . . . . . . . . . . . . . . . . . . . . . . . . . . . 44

STORY OF A LIFE . . . . . . . . . . . . . . . . . . . . . . . . . . 53
   Respect . . . . . . . . . . . . . . . . . . . . . . . . . . . . . . . . . . . 55
   Life on Mars . . . . . . . . . . . . . . . . . . . . . . . . . . . . . . 56
   Lord Randal . . . . . . . . . . . . . . . . . . . . . . . . . . . . . . . 59
   What About the Man? . . . . . . . . . . . . . . . . . . . . . . . 64
   An Old Man, a Crack Girl, and a Rat . . . . . . . . . . . 65
   Story of a Life . . . . . . . . . . . . . . . . . . . . . . . . . . . . . 70
   Presidential Debate . . . . . . . . . . . . . . . . . . . . . . . . 78

TROUBLED MAN . . . . . . . . . . . . . . . . . . . . . . . . . . . 81
   Troubled Man . . . . . . . . . . . . . . . . . . . . . . . . . . . . . 83
   Sound Mind . . . . . . . . . . . . . . . . . . . . . . . . . . . . . . 84
   Five White Men, a Blonde, and Jesus . . . . . . . . . . 88

Little Gods...........................................90
Jesus in Cedar Crest.................................93
Victor...............................................95
Restraints and the Voice.............................99

**RECOGNIZE** ....................................109
Girls...............................................111
Fidel...............................................112
No Kin of Mine......................................114
The Corner..........................................117
Mother..............................................119
Childhood...........................................121
French Fries........................................124
Social Club.........................................125
Recognize...........................................128
Sterling............................................129
Heroin..............................................131
Darkness............................................132

**BODY COUNT** ...................................133
Dead Man's Poker....................................135
Storm Inside the Calm...............................136
Asthma Code.........................................137
Gory Stories........................................145
Too Much Confusion..................................147
I Don't Want to Die.................................152
An Ordinary Head....................................153
Nicki Joyner........................................157
Body Count..........................................160

**BURNOUT** ......................................163
Booking Off.........................................165
Dead-icated.........................................166
Stress..............................................173
Meat in the Seat....................................176
Snowstorm...........................................177
Priorities..........................................178
Mean Streak.........................................179

# Contents

Roles. . . . . . . . . . . . . . . . . . . . . . . . . . . . . . . . . . . . . . . . . 182
State Card . . . . . . . . . . . . . . . . . . . . . . . . . . . . . . . . . . . . 183
Quit. . . . . . . . . . . . . . . . . . . . . . . . . . . . . . . . . . . . . . . . . . 184
Shit Rising. . . . . . . . . . . . . . . . . . . . . . . . . . . . . . . . . . . . . 185
Burnout . . . . . . . . . . . . . . . . . . . . . . . . . . . . . . . . . . . . . . . 188
Shame. . . . . . . . . . . . . . . . . . . . . . . . . . . . . . . . . . . . . . . . 189
Flat Line. . . . . . . . . . . . . . . . . . . . . . . . . . . . . . . . . . . . . . 193

**SHAMAN** . . . . . . . . . . . . . . . . . . . . . . . . . . . . . . . . . . 195
Reason . . . . . . . . . . . . . . . . . . . . . . . . . . . . . . . . . . . . . . . 197
Keep Hope Alive . . . . . . . . . . . . . . . . . . . . . . . . . . . . . . 198
Shaman . . . . . . . . . . . . . . . . . . . . . . . . . . . . . . . . . . . . . . 207
Payback . . . . . . . . . . . . . . . . . . . . . . . . . . . . . . . . . . . . . . 209
Rebecca . . . . . . . . . . . . . . . . . . . . . . . . . . . . . . . . . . . . . . 211
A Paramedic Again . . . . . . . . . . . . . . . . . . . . . . . . . . . . 224

**MEMORY** . . . . . . . . . . . . . . . . . . . . . . . . . . . . . . . . . . 237
Joe. . . . . . . . . . . . . . . . . . . . . . . . . . . . . . . . . . . . . . . . . . . 239
Snake Girl . . . . . . . . . . . . . . . . . . . . . . . . . . . . . . . . . . . . 241
Polish . . . . . . . . . . . . . . . . . . . . . . . . . . . . . . . . . . . . . . . . 243
Mr. and Mrs. Jones . . . . . . . . . . . . . . . . . . . . . . . . . . . . 245
Memory . . . . . . . . . . . . . . . . . . . . . . . . . . . . . . . . . . . . . . 247
Where Every Day Is Like Sunday . . . . . . . . . . . . . . . . . . 248
Reggie and Jill. . . . . . . . . . . . . . . . . . . . . . . . . . . . . . . . 250
You Ain't Fooling Me . . . . . . . . . . . . . . . . . . . . . . . . . . . 255
There Must Be a Mistake . . . . . . . . . . . . . . . . . . . . . . . . 256
Right There . . . . . . . . . . . . . . . . . . . . . . . . . . . . . . . . . . . 258
Flirt. . . . . . . . . . . . . . . . . . . . . . . . . . . . . . . . . . . . . . . . . . 259

**THE JOB** . . . . . . . . . . . . . . . . . . . . . . . . . . . . . . . . . . . 261
Thanks . . . . . . . . . . . . . . . . . . . . . . . . . . . . . . . . . . . . . . 263
Exeter . . . . . . . . . . . . . . . . . . . . . . . . . . . . . . . . . . . . . . . 266
Asthma. . . . . . . . . . . . . . . . . . . . . . . . . . . . . . . . . . . . . . 269
Change. . . . . . . . . . . . . . . . . . . . . . . . . . . . . . . . . . . . . . 272
Ups and Downs. . . . . . . . . . . . . . . . . . . . . . . . . . . . . . . 277
Last Day Together . . . . . . . . . . . . . . . . . . . . . . . . . . . . . 277
Life . . . . . . . . . . . . . . . . . . . . . . . . . . . . . . . . . . . . . . . . . 280
The Job. . . . . . . . . . . . . . . . . . . . . . . . . . . . . . . . . . . . . . 281

POSTSCRIPT . . . . . . . . . . . . . . . . . . . . . . . . . . . . . . . . . . . 284

ACKNOWLEDGMENTS . . . . . . . . . . . . . . . . . . . . . . . . . . 284

# Introduction

My name is Peter Canning. In *Paramedic: On the Front Lines of Medicine* I told how I left my job as an aide to the governor of Connecticut to become a paramedic on the city's streets and how I struggled in my first year to prove myself worthy of the job. This book *Rescue 471: A Paramedic's Stories* continues my story over the next three years as I battle with life and death, and mature into a seasoned medic, confident of my skills and abilities but smart enough to know there is always more to learn and overcome. I have just turned forty; my partner for much of the time period of the book, Arthur Gasparrini, is in his early fifties. While there are other medics of my age—and a few of Arthur's—working in the city today, emergency medical services (EMS) is largely a young person's field. The physical demands of the job aside, burnout is a common occupational hazard for paramedics, particuarly those in an urban setting, cutting short many promising careers. High call volume, continual exposure to death and serious injury, and the incredible abuse of the 911 system gradually wear at your sanity. These stresses and pressures of the job eventually caused me to come perilously close to losing my way. I almost forgot the most important of lessons: that the focus of your work is on your patient, the person that you are helping, and that you can't let anything—stress, frustration, fatigue—come between you, your patient, and the very best care you can give, medical and emotional. This book tells how I battled burnout and found renewal in this work I love. Here are the sights, sounds, and emotions of the job: the flurry of action in critical moments and the hard loyalty of tested partners. While there is plenty of lights-and-sirens action, the job encompasses so much more. Here also is a view of children in peril, the aged facing death, troubled minds trying to cope with a difficult world, and the heroism of those who keep dreaming and loving in spite of the harshness of their world. These are my stories and theirs. They are all true. A few of the stories have been resequenced. Some names and details have been altered to protect confidentiality.

# ARTHUR

*Spending forty hours a week in an ambulance with the same person, month after month, year after year, is a lot like being married. Sometimes you get along great; other times you can't stand each other. You are fiercely loyal in the big picture.*

# Kools

Our ambulance 471 is dispatched for a man not breathing. My partner, Arthur Gasparrini, races us through Hartford's downtown business district. He brakes hard at Main and Church, as cars oblivious to our whirling lights and sirens continue through the intersection. Arthur slams the air horn, then hurtles us on north up Main Street, past decaying public housing, abandoned apartment buildings, and businesses with bars on their windows.

Ahead, by a Spanish supermarket, a man with wild matted hair runs out into the street and flags us down. "Four-seven-one arrival," I tell the dispatcher.

When I step out I can smell the brakes smoking. I grab my equipment from the ambulance's side door.

"Come quick," the man says. "My buddy fell out."

We follow him a short way down the street, then up a muddy embankment and around the side of a boarded-up apartment building.

A man is lying facedown in the weeds. We quickly roll him over. There is a vomit on his chin and the front of his shirt. His body is cool. I put my hand on his chest. A shudder, then no movement. I put my fingers on his neck. "He's still got a pulse." I look at his pupils.

"Pinpoint?" Arthur says.

I nod. Pinpoint. A likely heroin overdose.

Arthur gets out the ambu-bag and applies the plastic face mask to the man's face. He squeezes the bag, forcing air through the mask into the man's mouth and down into his lungs, breathing for him.

3

"He ain't dead, is he?" The man who called us stands over my shoulder.

"Not yet. Is he your friend?" I ask.

"No, no, he's just an acquaintance."

The man has thick track marks on his arms, scarring from years of shooting up. "He did heroin today?" I ask.

"No, I mean maybe, yeah, yeah, he did. Like I said, he's just an acquaintance."

I find a small vein in his right arm and insert a catheter. Blood returns into the needle's chamber. I attach a small rubber IV port to the back of the catheter.

"Is he going to be all right?"

With a syringe I draw two milligrams of Narcan out of a small vial. Narcan is an antiopiate that quickly reverses the effects of heroin. I inject the drug through the IV port. I'm worried we might be a little late with this guy.

"Any sign of breathing yet?" I ask. Thirty seconds have passed.

Arthur stops bagging. Still no movement. He resumes bagging. I'm starting to get a little anxious.

I draw up another two milligrams and give him the extra dose.

When another minute passes and still no effect, I say, "I'm going to tube him."

"Do you want to wait a little more?"

"He looks pretty out."

I am in charge on all our calls (as an EMT-Paramedic I am more highly trained than Arthur, who is an EMT-Intermediate), but I usually give weight to his suggestions. He has a good point about giving the Narcan more time to work, but I think this man may be too far gone, and I like to be aggressive when it comes to gaining a better airway for a patient.

I take my intubation kit out of the blue bag and switch places with Arthur so I can be at the head. Holding the laryngoscope in my left hand, I slide the steel blade into the man's mouth, then I sweep the tongue out of the way and lift up. The small lightbulb on the end of the blade illuminates the throat. I see my target: the narrow opening between the white vocal cords that guard the entrance to the windpipe. If I miss, I end up in the stomach. I pass the tube through the cords. "I'm in."

Arthur attaches the ambu-bag to the tube. With my stethoscope, I listen under each armpit, hearing lung sounds as Arthur squeezes the bag. Then I listen over the stomach. No sounds. Perfect. "Let's get him out of here," I say.

"We have a problem," Arthur says.

"What?"

The man's eyes are open.

"Whoa!" Before I can stop him, he grabs the tube.

"No, hold on!"

He yanks it out of his throat, sits bolt upright, and pukes over himself, then turns onto all four and pukes again. "Goddamn," he moans.

I shake my head at Arthur's grin.

The man looks around: at me, at Arthur, at the guy standing with us. "Fuck."

"You okay?" his friend asks.

"No, I'm not okay."

"I thought you was dead," he says.

"Dead, bullshit, I ain't dead. What'd you fucking do to me?" He gets shakily to his feet.

"I was trying to help your sorry ass."

The man pats his shirt pocket, then pats it again harder and looks down to see it empty.

"Where's my cigarettes? Who took my cigarettes? Shit. Did you take my cigarettes? Where's my Kools?"

"Never mind your cigarettes," I say. "You should come to the hospital with us."

"I ain't going nowhere." He notices the IV plug in his arm.

He rips it out as I weakly say, "Don't."

"Fuck this shit." He pats his pants pockets. "Where's my money? You took my money? Somebody robbed me!"

"We didn't take your money," I say. "You weren't breathing. You need to come to the hospital. What I gave you may wear off before the heroin leaves your system."

"Heroin? I didn't do any heroin. What are you talking about? I'm breathing fine. Did you jump me, motherfucker?"

"No, man, you just done fellout."

"What'd you call the cops for?"

"We're not cops."

"You some kind of friend," he says. "You some kind of friend calling the law. Fuck you, fuck all of you." He scowls and walks away.

"You're welcome," Arthur says, as the man disappears behind the overgrown hedges.

"How's that for thanks?" his friend says. "How's that for thanks?"

We start gathering up our gear, the IV wrappers, intubation equipment.

The man lights a cigarette, still shaking his head.

I note the brand when he puts the pack back in his pocket. "Kools?" I say.

"I prefer Camels," he says. "But Kools'll do me."

# Arthur

Arthur is a nudist. "Show them your tan line," I say. He takes off his watch and reveals the white underneath that stands out against his deeply browned skin.

"I wouldn't kid you," I say. "There's the living proof. That's his only line. Tell them about it, Arthur."

Nurses don't know what to think, and they listen with interest and mild disbelief as Arthur talks about the campground where he and his wife go every weekend. He plays naked tennis and naked volleyball and drinks iced tea naked in the Bare Bottoms Bar. He says it is like skinny-dipping all the time. They have all ages, shapes, and sizes there. It is a wholesome family environment. Once when he and his wife invited me over for dinner, I saw on his refrigerator a Christmas card sent by a family he knows from the campground. The father, mother, and five children sit on a bench in descending order, bare backsides to the camera, heads turned, waving.

Before I worked with Arthur, I thought he was a nice, laid-back, type B personality, a friendly guy with a smile and warm words for everyone. He used to be Shawn Kinkade's partner, but he switched to me because I work a better schedule. Shawn works Monday through Wednesday six A.M. to six P.M. I work Tuesday through Thursday seven A.M. to seven P.M., which are the same days of the week Arthur's wife works as a hairdresser. By working with me, they get an extra day a week at the campground and he gets to sleep an hour later in the morning. When he became my partner, I joked with Shawn, handing him a Snickers bar in return for Arthur.

"He's a good partner," Shawn said as we shook on the deal. "A nice guy. Good luck." He smiled.

"Good luck?" I got a sudden queasy feeling.

I am glad to be working with Arthur. He is strong, knows the city, has a good work ethic, and likes to drive. It is the driving, however, that people have warned me about.

"He's a maniac," one says.

"After Glenn," I say, referring to my last partner, a young man who drove like a cowboy on a mustang chasing Indians, "he can't be too bad."

No response.

"Can he?"

A smile.

In the city, cars don't respect ambulances. They don't pull over. They either keep going or stop suddenly in the middle of the road. If they do pull over, they pull to the left, not the right, and usually the pullover is a sudden swerve in front of you. They don't know the traffic laws, play music too loud, talk on cellular phones, are more interested in people walking along the sidewalk than cars on the street, are zombies, think they own the road, or just don't care. And they get away with it. I have never seen a car pulled over and a driver lectured—much less ticketed—for failing to yield to an emergency vehicle. At worst, drivers get a frustrated EMT slamming the air horn at them and shaking a fist. Not only does bad driving delay our emergency response, it is a real safety threat.

Arthur, I learn on the very first day, can't stand for cars to disrespect our ambulance when we are running lights and sirens. He races up on traffic, blasting the air horn above the modulating double sirens. If the car ahead of us won't pull over, he swears and jams his finger down on the air horn button as if the sound itself will explode them off the road. When the car finally pulls over, he often slows, glares, and gestures at the driver. You idiot. Moron.

We're racing down Main Street. Arthur is right on the tail of a black sedan with tinted windows that won't pull over. He slams the horn.

"Arthur," I say.

The car doesn't yield.

"Arthur," I say.

He hits the air horn again, still close on the car's bumper.

"Arthur, our turn was back there."

I adopt the same policy I had with Glenn. I strap on my seat belt and pray we will make it to the scene alive. I say nothing about his driving. My bargain with the devil is I let my partners do most of the to-scene driving. Because I am six-eight, my legs are cramped in the driver's seat. I prefer the passenger side while we wait for a call. I fold my legs up and set them on the dashboard while I read. The passenger seat is also nice for arriving on an accident or other scene. I can jump right out and not have to worry about where to park. Also, the less I drive, the less likely I am to have an accident, which would threaten the $150 year-end bonus they give to those of us with perfect driving records, but I don't tell this to Arthur, nor will I give him a cut of my bonus. What I do tell him when we are en route to the hospital is to go on a three, no lights, no sirens. It is rare that I will ask for a two, lights and sirens, and extremely so that I ask for a one, lights and sirens in a serious hurry. I need to work in the back of the ambulance and I cannot work when I am being thrown all over and subjected to sudden stops and violent air horns. Unless the patient is gunshot or needs a surgeon immediately or has an injury or sickness I simply can't handle, the nonemergency mode works fine. It makes no sense to me to race lights and sirens to the ER, then wait in triage ten minutes or more for a room assignment, and then have the patient wait even longer in the room to be seen first by a nurse, then a doctor. Time to hospital does not equal time to treatment. If I can provide the treatment, I do it in my ambulance. The emergency is then usually over. No need to risk our lives rushing through traffic.

"Go on a three," I say.

Spending forty hours a week in an ambulance with the same person, month after month, year after year, is a lot like being married. Sometimes you get along great, other times you can't stand each other. You are fiercely loyal in the big picture, but you can often be a petty complainer about the small stuff to anyone who will listen.

There are some days I come home and I think I just can't deal with Arthur anymore. "He's a psychopath, a complete maniac," I'll say.

And I am sure he feels the same about me. I picture him at home, saying, "What an asshole my partner is. He doesn't respect me. Always yelling at me. He doesn't know how good he's got it."

It is true I yell at him when we do a hairy call, constantly telling him to do three things at once. "Get him on the monitor. I need that bag spiked. No, no, give me that thing. I need the thing. Now!"

"What thing?"

"The thing, the thing, you know."

"Help me out."

"The thing you use to, you know, squeeze air, the . . . the . . ."

"The ambu-bag."

"Yeah, yeah, give it to me!"

Sometimes, probably not often enough, I go up to him afterward and say, "Arthur, I'm sorry. Like I told you when we started working together, if I am yelling at you, I am really yelling at myself, so don't take it personally. You did a great job on that call. You are a good partner."

"Thank you," he says, with a hint of understated righteousness.

I do work him hard and don't compliment him nearly as often as I should. I don't know why that is. Maybe it is because he is older, and I want to believe that I can still work at his age, that I will not complain about being tired, that I will be every bit as fit as the twenty-five-year-olds who make up the bulk of our company, that I will always be strong, a good worker. If I compliment him too much he may slow up, take it easier. I want us both to be supermen.

I know there are many things I do that irritate Arthur, particularly when I am tired from working overtime shifts. I know I should thank him more, but I find it difficult to do. What he hates most about me, I think, is when I am grumpy or don't talk to him. There are some mornings I just want to get on the road and be left alone. I don't want to hear about his weekend at the campground, whether or not he won his naked tennis match, or about the naked yard work he did on his trailer lot at the camp. Nothing against him—sometimes I just don't want to talk to anyone, I don't want to be there. The misanthrope that is close to my center becomes a big hairy ape that sits in the shotgun seat, swatting down all attempts at conversation and good humor.

I always come in early and check out my gear and the rig, so when he arrives on the dot of seven, we are ready to go. "Let me just check the oil," he says.

"But Arthur," I say, "they serviced the car last night. Let's get on the road."

"You can never be sure," he says.

If we're down a quart, I have to wait for him to go over to the garage, where he spends fifteen minutes talking about cars with the mechanics. Meanwhile, I'm impatient to get out on the road, worried I am going to miss saving a life or delivering a baby. Later when the company sends out a memo about crews being subject to suspension or firing if the oil runs out, as it has in two other rigs, I say nothing to Arthur, though I know if there were two of me in the crew we'd never check the oil, and probably end up blowing up the engine and getting fired.

I buy a paper every morning. He insists on paying for half of it, handing me a quarter. It takes me five minutes to read the paper. I just skim the headlines and the few articles that look interesting. It takes him all day to read the paper. And he is always reading the paper aloud to me when I am trying to read a book, and worse, he will read the paper in the form of a question that demands an answer. "So what, did they discover life on Mars they're saying here?"

"Yup," I'll say.

"Huh?"

"Yes, they did."

"What was it, some kind of microscopic bacteria?"

"I don't know."

"It was. Microscopic bacteria. I'll be damned. Who would have thunk it?"


On Albany Avenue, as we race to an unknown, people hold their hands over their ears as we pass. Ahead, three large young men in baggy clothing saunter in front of the ambulance. Arthur slams the brakes and shouts "Get out of the road!" He shakes his fist.

They glare and make hand gestures at us, which I fear are gang signs for I'm going to put a cap in your ass.

"Arthur," I say, "you are going to get shot one of these days."

"They were on your side," he says.

"Oh, thanks," I say.


Arthur listens to the oldies station on the radio. I love all this music, but when you hear "Green-Eyed Lady," "Brandy," "Brown Sugar," and "In the Still of the Night," every day, twelve hours a day, three days a week, every month of every year, it all becomes elevator music. I complain, then he'll switch to a classic rock station, and then I get tired of "Layla" and "Sweet Home Alabama." Every now and then while he's inside writing his run form, I'll switch to rap or modern rock head-banging music, just to mess with him. Later he'll surreptitiously turn the volume down or change the channel. Sometimes when he gets out of the car, I'll do the same, turning the oldies music off or just putting the volume all the way down. An hour later he'll turn the radio on and inch the volume up, never saying anything about it having been turned off, turned down, or the station switched.

Every night at six-thirty, he calls up dispatch and asks if we can come in off the road. "My honey's cooking dinner tonight," he'll say. Every night his wife is cooking him something special for dinner. I want to do extra calls, I want the extra pay. But no. Six-thirty comes along, he calls up dispatch and asks if we can come in for the crew change because his honey is cooking him something special for dinner. And because he is nice, they most always let us come in, while they keep other "honeyless" crews out long past their crew change.

"You are robbing my retirement savings," I say as we head in. "When I am old and destitute, I will curse you. No six-packs of Ensure in my minirefrigerator. I'll have to recycle my Depends."

"Tough luck. My honey's got dinner on the stove."

Sometimes I don't mind going in. After a long day I'm beat and I can use the beer waiting for me at home. If I'm in a good mood I'll turn the volume up on the radio when we're heading in, and we'll sing along to the oldies. "Chantilly Lace." And a pretty face. Hot day. "Summer in the City."

For all his idiosyncrasies, Arthur is a very good partner. He is solid, reliable, strong. He never complains when I decide we need to carry a patient down a flight of stairs instead of making them walk. He does what I ask, even when I am shouting at him to do three things at once. And even though he is six-two, he always lets me take the back of the stretcher so I don't have to be bent over like Quasimodo, pulling the front. And for all our spats and silent feuding, we have a good time together.

I hate going into nursing homes, but with Arthur it can be fun. "Let's get the old folks stirred up," he says as we enter the front door. The old people are always lining the corridors in their wheelchairs. As we roll down the hall, Arthur has something to say to each of them.

"Hello, young lady!" he says to an old woman in a wheelchair, her head down.

She looks up, surprised, and breaks into a big smile. "Well, hello."

"What a lovely sweater you're wearing! I'd like to find one like that for my honey."

"Thank you."

To a man wearing an army veteran's hat: "General!" He salutes. "Top of the morning to you. Everything shipshape?"

The man returns the salute. "That's right."

He continues this way down the hall. "What pretty white heads," he says to the assembled ladies in their wheelchairs. "It must be beauty parlor day." The smiles break out like falling dominoes as we pass.

Ahead an old man in a wheelchair barrels out of a room, causing us to stop suddenly to avoid him. "Out of my way, out of my way," he grumbles at us as he motors past.

"That's going to be you in twenty years," I say.

"Maybe," Arthur says, "except I'll be naked."

Our patient is an old lady who fractured her hand in a fall. She is very anxious. "Don't worry, we won't drop you," he says, "not like that last lady."

"What!"

"We never drop anyone on Wednesday."

"It's Thursday."

"Whoops. I mean, we shouldn't be saying whoops, that's what we said the last time. A bad word in this business."

"You dropped someone?"

"Right on her head. I mean we're not supposed to be talking

about it, advice of lawyers. But she's not feeling any pain, at least not anymore, poor dear."

By the time we leave, he has her laughing and comfortable, her mind at ease. As we head back down the corridor, the troops have their eyes raised, ready to converse as we wheel back past. Arthur smiles, laughs, and jokes with all of them.

Later in the day, we take a patient from Saint Francis Hospital back to a nursing home after a ten-day stay for congestive heart failure. He goes through the same routine with the residents in the hallway, making their day.

"A little encouragement means the world to these people," a nurse says to Arthur as we leave. "You can see it."

When we get back outside, he says, "If I ever end up in one of these places, put a bullet in my brain."


# Rescue 471


The 911 call comes from a nursing home for an unconscious patient. The sixty-one-year-old man is lying on his bed with his mouth open. His color is good. His respiratory rate is fine. He has a strong, steady pulse; his blood pressure is a little high, but not dangerously so. I open his eyelids to check his pupils. He tries to roll his eyes back into his head.

The nurse tells me he has a history of seizures, but no one saw him have one this morning. I listen to his lungs with a stethoscope. The man holds his breath. When I move my stethoscope away, he resumes breathing.

I take his hand and hold it in the air above his face. I let it go. It lands safely away from his face; he's conscious. A faker.

I break open an ammonia inhalant and hold it under his

nose. Again he tries to hold his breath. "You've got to breathe sometime," I say.

After about thirty seconds, he finally has to breathe and moves his head to avoid the smell.

I look at his feet. I am tempted to tickle their bottoms.

"Does he do this often?" I ask the nurse.

"No, but he's been giving us a lot of trouble the last couple days. He's been very difficult, very agitated about being here."

"You want us to take him to the hospital."

"Yeah, I wouldn't want anything to happen."

At the hospital, I tell the triage nurse we were called for an unconscious man, whom we believe to be faking. She gets out a box of ammonia inhalants and does the same routine I did.

After twenty seconds, the man is moving his head away. The nurse looks disgusted. She calls down to the ER and tells them we're bringing down a guy feigning unresponsiveness.

We put him on a gurney in the hall, where they can watch him.

We're dispatched to a drunk, then a moment later, the dispatcher says, "Four-seven-one, disregard. Go to Enfield Street for a shooting. A man shot in the leg."

Arthur hits the lights, and does a U-turn on Main Street. I put on my gloves and lay my trauma shears on the dashboard.

We arrive at the address before the cops. I get out the $O_2$ bag, and we wait behind the ambulance as the first cruiser pulls in. The cop gets out, hand on his holster, and nods to us. We follow him up the steps of the house. He bangs on the door, then steps to the side. I wince at the thought of a shotgun blast blowing a hole in the door.

The door is slightly ajar; he pushes it open and shouts, "Police."

A voice beckons us in, and we follow the cop as he moves in slowly, ready to draw.

An old man is sitting in a decrepit armchair.

"Somebody shot in here?"

"No, no, I don't believe so."

"We got a report of a shooting."

"Hmm, wait a minute. David!" he calls into the other room, "David, come out here!"

I expect to see his son, a tough young male, with a bloody leg, limp out. Instead, another old man appears and says, "I called the police. I got shot. Look here."

The man does not appear wounded. He is pointing down to his ankle. I have him sit in a chair so I can examine him. I remove a dirty black sneaker and a sock. There is not a mark on his foot.

"Where did you get shot?" I ask.

"Right here, right here is where it hurts." He points to the lateral side of his left ankle. There is no wound.

"There's nothing wrong with you," Arthur says. "How much have you had to drink?"

"A couple of beers and some brandy. But I got hit, I tell you."

The cop cancels his backup unit.

"You didn't get shot," I say.

"I was walking down the street and something hit me. If I didn't get shot, then something hit me. Take me to the hospital now and get it checked out."

I remove the other sneaker and compare both feet. They look the same. The only difference is, he is complaining of pain when I press one spot on the left ankle.

"Take me to the hospital, I tell you."

"There's nothing wrong with you."

"I got hit, I tell you, officer."

"I should arrest you for making a false complaint," the officer says.

"But, I got hit, I got hit."

"All right, then, let's go," I say.


"Once again four-seven-one to the rescue," Arthur says as we clear the hospital.


We do a motor vehicle accident (MVA) out on Edgewood Street. It is minor and we transport only one patient, who says he has back pain. Insuranceitis, as Arthur calls it. At Saint

Francis, the old guy from the nursing home is still on the stretcher in the hallway, nobody paying him any mind.

We're called to a market in the north end for back pain. A cop leads us into a back storage room, where the temperature is nearly 120. A young man is sitting on the ground, sweat dripping off him. His hands are bound behind him with twine.

"He says his back hurts," the cop says.

"My back, my head. Goddamn, I can't move," the man shouts.

"What's wrong?" I ask.

"They all beating the crap out of me. That's what's wrong. Feel my head. That's what's wrong."

"Who was beating you?"

"The three of them."

The three are the store's owners. They shake their heads and laugh. "He was moving fine till you came. He was trying to get away."

"They were hitting me with shovels, man," he says. "Feel my head."

I look around but don't see any shovels. I feel his head. He has a small hematoma on it. There are some welts on his back.

"You let me go, I show you were they hit me."

The sweat is pouring off both of us now. I tell Arthur we need to C-spine him.

"I don't care what you do to me. You get me to the hospital. I could be dying. I think I got internal bleeding."

I come back with the stretcher and long board to find the cop releasing the man from his bonds. Then she handcuffs him.

"He can't be cuffed," I say. "We have to put him on the board."

"I can't undo him," she says.

"Why not?"

"I don't have the key."

"You don't have the key?" I say.

"I didn't think I was going to be arresting anyone today," she says.

"You didn't? Well, where is the key?"

"At the station house."

Arthur and I look at each other. We are both sweating profusely. We look at the guy, who is dripping water.

"I'm dying here, man," the guy says. "You all just letting me die. I know I got internal bleeding."

The cop radios her base and learns that an officer stationed at the hospital up the street has a key.

"Let's just put him on the stretcher," I say.

We finally get him out to the ambulance and he jabbers the whole way.

I take his vital signs, which are fine. The guy won't give me his name. I sit there toweling the sweat off my forehead while Arthur drives the few blocks to the hospital.

"How you doing?" I say to our patient.

"I can't breathe," he says. He starts puffing and panting.

"How long were you knocked out for?"

"Two, three minutes. That's at a minimum."

"No kidding."

"I think I got internal bleeding," he says.

"Did he say he had eternal bleeding?" Arthur asks when I get back in the ambulance.

"He said *internal*."

"It sounded like *eternal*. I think you're just giving him more credit than he's due. Like the lady who took motowns and peanut butter balls."

We both laugh. It is funny the things that either people misstate or you mishear. Motrin and phenobarbital become motowns and peanut butter balls. Alzheimer's disease becomes old-timer's disease. A cyst becomes a sister. The best one I ever heard was from another medic—a patient told him his uncle had died of a massive fart. The doctor had probably said he died of a massive infarction of the heart, and the poor guy misunderstood and believed the uncle had died from a giant fart blowing up inside him.

"Maybe he did say *eternal*," I say.

"He did. I tell you, he did," Arthur says. "I got eternal bleeding."

\* \* \*

We clear the hospital and get sent right off for a leg fracture on Garden Street. It is a rundown house. Four men sit on third-hand couches watching a tiny black-and-white TV. On the wall someone has drawn a large picture of a Rastafarian smoking a giant spliff. LORD OF LORDS, KINGS OF KINGS is written next to it. They are all drinking beer. The man whose leg hurts is in his fifties; the others in their thirties. We look at the ankle; it looks barely swollen. He says it's been bothering him for about two months now, mon.

"Make sure dey get X rays," one of the men says. "He get him some crutches so he get himself around."

"They'll X-ray it, but I don't know if they'll give him crutches. It don't look broken to me," Arthur says.

"They give me crutches when I just twist my ankle," one man says. "Ask for them. They got 'em dere."

We take him to Mount Sinai and leave him in the waiting room.

As soon as we get back in our ambulance, the Hartford police dispatcher calls us. "Four-seven-one respond to Maple Street for a firefighter injured—high fall. On a one."

We both swear. We're deep north and the address on Maple is deep south. And it's rush hour.

We go flying across town against the traffic. I am thinking this is the big one. The guy fell off a building and I'm going to have to tube him. The firefighters are going to be all over us to help their buddy. We're going to have to be quick. Get him tubed, get him C-spined, and get out of there.

These are the calls that if you do great, you're a hero; you fuck up, every firefighter in the state will be on your case.

When we arrive, three ladder trucks are in the road. The air is heavy with smoke. I grab the green bag and head into the scene while Arthur pulls the stretcher and readies the C-spine gear.

I walk through the trucks and see several groups of fire-fighters with soot-blackened faces. No one is hailing me. I look around to see who's in charge. "Where's the guy who fell?" I ask. They look at me blankly. Finally one says, "There's your man over there."

He points to a group of five firefighters, all in full turnout gear. They are all standing. I look around as if I'm missing something. "Where?" I say.

"Right there. That man."

A young guy steps forward. "I fell on my shoulder," he says.

"How far?"

"Length of my body."

"Did you hit your head?"

"Just my shoulder."

I stand there and say nothing for a moment, then: "Okay, the ambulance is this way."

"I'll come get you later," one firefighter says to him.

"Yeah, okay."

Arthur is just coming into the crowd now, pushing the stretcher with the long boards on it, along with head rolls, belts, and a C-collar, and he is shocked to see me walking back.

"This is him," I say. "Fell about five feet on his shoulder. Didn't hit his head."

I throw the green bag in the side door and go around to the driver's seat. Arthur slowly puts the board away, then has the man get in on the bench. He splints his shoulder. From what I hear, it sounds like his shoulder popped out of the joint, then popped back in. He has some elbow pain, too, but nothing seems broken. I imagine some firefighter calling 911 and making up a big bad story to get his buddy an ambulance quicker. I tell the dispatcher we're on an easy three to Hartford. I know all the other ambulances were sitting waiting to see how quick we'd leave the scene and on what priority. A one would have been the big bad one; a two would have been significant enough to ask about later—probably a head injury, some signs of shock—a three, nothing; an easy three—bullshit.

When we get to the hospital, the guy doesn't want to be wheeled in a chair, which is what we usually offer for an injury or a drunk when we haven't used the stretcher. But he's a tough guy, and he walks in, arm splinted, carrying his helmet and coat in the other hand. I don't even bother to go in. Arthur gives the report.

We clear and they send us on a priority two to an unknown all the way down Franklin Avenue. It turns out to be a six-year-old who fell, and one of her front baby teeth is sticking out at a ninety-degree angle to the other. Her mother is all upset that the tooth needs to be fixed.

We are speechless. "Why did you call us?" I say. "I mean, what do you want us to do?"

"Fix it," she says.

"It's a baby tooth. It's going to fall out on its own."

"But she can't eat with it like this."

I kneel down and look at it. I am thinking about just grabbing it and yanking it out. I touch it and wobble it a little. The girl starts to cry and hides her head in her mom's waist. She looks at me like I am a villain.

"There's nothing we can do, and they're not going to be able to do anything at the hospital. Does she have a dentist? Take her to the dentist. This isn't an emergency. I mean, we'll be happy to drive you to the hospital, but really we wouldn't be anything but a taxi service."

She says nothing.

"You could tie a piece of string around it, and the other end to a door, and then yank the door open," I say.

She looks at me like she doesn't understand what I am saying and hugs her daughter tighter to her.

Arthur and I look at each other and shake our heads.

"What kind of insurance do you have?" I ask.

"State," she says.

"Do you have an HMO?"

She shakes her head no.

"In the future," I say, "you will have to contact the gate-keeper at your HMO, and they will say no way will they pay for a loose tooth to be transported in an ambulance, and it will cost you personally two hundred dollars if you go."

She looks at me with fear.

"But right now," I say, "the state will pay for it. Two hundred dollars. It's up to you. They won't be able to do anything for her. You're just going to sit in the waiting room, but if you want to go we'll take you."

She looks at her daughter, who is looking up at her, and then she looks at us.

"What'll it be?"

She looks back at her daughter. She gives her a hug. "We'll go," she says.

I shake my head, then say, "Well, let's get going."

Hartford Hospital is busy. They have a major trauma going in room one. The triage nurse looks at us like we are kidding her when we give the report. She looks at the girl's tooth and then looks at the mother. She sends them to the waiting room. "If we keep them out there long enough, maybe it will fall out on its own," she says.

Our last 911 call is for a man with a swollen hand. He meets us at the curb. I look at his hand, then ask him which hospital he wants to go to. Saint Francis. "Okay. Get in." I get his name, birth date, address, and state card number as we drive.

As we're walking in to Saint Francis, I see the guy with "eternal bleeding" being walked to a squad car, hands cuffed behind him, headed for a night behind bars. "I'm going to sue, I'm going to sue," he is shouting at the officer. "I could be dying!"

"Yeah, yeah, yeah," the officer says, as he opens the back door for him. "Watch your head."

In the ER I see the guy from the nursing home still on the stretcher, but this time a doctor is examining him. "You may have had a seizure," the doctor, a moonlighter who has just come on duty, says. He is reading the nursing home report. "That's why the convalescent home sent you here. Do you remember that?"

The man has a sour look on his face. "I want something to eat," he says.

# Kids

Arthur and I compete to see who can get the biggest smiles from kids. He, the grandfather, usually wins out, particularly with the babies. This despite my monkey imitations, which are widely acclaimed and always draw a positive response from the simian inmates when I visit the Central Park Zoo. "It's not that they like you better," I say. "It's just that you've had more practice. Like since George Washington was president and pterodactyls flew in the sky."

"Jealousy will get you nowhere," he says, lifting the baby up over his head, smiling and saying, "You're an adorable little muffin, yes, you are." And they giggle and smile and laugh.

"Please," I say. I hold my hands out to take the baby.

"Stand back," he says, "you might scare her."

We often introduce ourselves to kids as Fred and Barney or Mufasa and Riffiki. If they speak Spanish I will call Arthur *un perro viejo*, an old dog. *"Feo, tonto, gordo,"* I'll say. Ugly, dumb, fat. And they will laugh, holding their hands to their mouths to try to keep it in.

"What's that?" Arthur will say.

"I told them you were very handsome, strong, and bright."

"Why do I get the feeling you just insulted me?"

*"Muy tonto,"* I'll say. Very dumb.

And they'll laugh again.

Arthur is a good sport about it.

Sometimes we introduce ourselves as father and son. "He's my dad," I'll say.

"That's right, son," Arthur will say.

We will be standing by a fish tank. "In Norway, where we come from," Arthur will say, "we eat fish alive."

"No," the kids will say, laughing.

"Swallow them whole."

"Don't they squirm?"

"That's the best part," Arthur will say, "but they don't squirm for long."

A pediatrician from the Connecticut Children's Medical Center (CCMC) rides with us one day. Arthur says it must be hard working with kids who are so sick. The doctor says it can be hard, but the thing with kids is they often get better, and when they are sick, it is rarely their fault. Adults, on the other hand, are usually sick because of their own lifestyle choices—heavy eating, lack of exercise, smoking, alcohol, violence. And in the end, adults all die.

Neither of us likes doing calls where the kid is either seriously ill or seems to be seriously hurt. "What a shame," Arthur says when we finish a long-distance transfer for a kid with leukemia. "Nice kid. Nice family."

Kids are hard, hard emotionally and hard medically. They are not little adults. They are a completely different category. It's much harder to tell how sick they are. Sometimes they are much frailer; other times their resilience will surprise you.

A three-year-old girl, left unattended by her mother, falls thirty feet out of an open window and lands on cement. A bystander picks her up and says she is not breathing. The first EMTs on scene, Faith Creer and Cindy Hudson, call for a medic. The girl is unconscious, they say, and only breathing sporadically. Arthur and I arrive and break through the crowd. While we C-spine the child on a half board, I get out an ambu-bag and assist respirations. She stops breathing and is out of it completely, but after a few breaths of the ambu-bag, she opens her eyes, breathes, then conks back out. On the radio, I call Hartford Hospital, requesting the trauma room. We're two minutes out. I am bagging the unresponsive girl as we come through the door. The room is full of adults in medical gowns, expecting the worst. "Fell thirty feet, landed on cement, breathing very erratic." As I say this the little girl opens her eyes and looks around.

"You sure it was thirty feet onto cement?" the doctor says. Other than an abrasion on her forehead, she doesn't have a scratch on her body.

"Yes, and her breathing was very erratic, like periods of apnea," I say.

They are *goo-goo*ing and *gaa-gaa*ing her now. She is wide awake. The doctor is looking at me like I am some excited rookie who misread the scene. They do a complete workup, and all they find is a hematoma on her liver. On the news that night, they interview local residents, who describe the fall and how she wasn't breathing when they picked her up. They also say this wasn't the first time she'd been left alone.

Two days later we are up in Windsor when we get a call to a day care center where a two-year-old fell two feet and hit her head. She has a little bump but is otherwise fine and peacefully reading a book. They have called her mother, who is on her way there. She wants her daughter seen at CCMC. I tell Art to get a backboard and C-collar equipment. While I am writing down the information the day care teacher is giving me about the girl, I look over at her. Suddenly her eyes do a little roll, her head falls to the side, and she conks out. I grab her hand and give her a little pinch. Nothing. No reaction. I open her eyes, and they do not react at all. I look out the window. Art is kneeling down by the ambulance, trying to get a kitten to come to him. He is going, "Here, kitty, kitty, kitty. Here, kitty, kitty, kitty." I bang on the window. He pays no attention. I bang again. Hard. He glances up at me. Let's go, I mouth.

The girl is completely out of it. We C-spine her quickly, put an oxygen mask on, and are wheeling her out just as the mother comes in. "This is all precautionary," I say. We get her in the back of the ambulance and I tell Arthur to go on a two, lights and sirens. The call has me puzzled. The girl didn't fall two feet. She was fine and then boom, she was out of it. I do a terrible thing then. When someone is faking, I hold their hand over their head and drop it. If they are faking, the hand conveniently misses their face. If they are not, it smacks them. I usually only do it when I think they might be faking. I hold her hand over her head and release it. It smacks her hard right in the nose. She doesn't stir. I put a tourniquet on her arm and stick her with a 22 IV. She doesn't flinch. I radio Children's. Unresponsive two-year-old. Fell two feet. Was fine, then boom. Out cold. Just as we come into the city, Arthur hits a bump. The car goes airborne and hits the road hard. The girl opens her eyes. "Mommy," she says.

Her mother turns around in the seat. "Katie."

"Mommy," Katie says.

Moments later when we wheel her into the hospital, she is smiling and talking like a normal two-year-old. "Look," I say to the doctor, "I know what she looks like now, and I'm telling you kids confuse the hell of out me, but she was out cold. Completely. I know she's fine now. I'm just telling you, her eyes rolled back and she went out."

The doctor nods and smiles. They keep her for observation for four hours and send her home with a clean bill of health.


A couple of months later, we are transporting a four-year-old boy who banged his head on a table and, according to the mother, is sleepy and isn't acting like himself. He doesn't seem quite right to me either. Again, we go lights and sirens. Just to be safe. At Children's, the nurse is also bothered, as the child keeps closing his eyes and doesn't respond to pinches. "Let's get a doctor in here," she calls to another nurse. The doctor comes in, looks at the kid, then pinches his belly—hard. The kid lets out a bloodcurdling scream. The nurses look at the doctor like he's a villain; they're also upset he has belittled their diagnosis. "Hey, you just have to use a little force," he says. "Can't CAT scan everyone."

The kid stays awake for the rest of his visit, screaming every time the doctor walks by the door to his room.

"I'll let you try that next time we have a kid with a possible head injury," I say to Arthur. "Just give him a vicious pinch in the belly."

"I don't think so," he says. "You're the paramedic. It's what you get the big bucks for."

# SAVING LIVES

*I always want to be perfect; it's what people expect from medical professionals. However, like most everything in life, you never bat a thousand. You don't like to think that you can come up short.*

# Perfect

My old paramedic preceptor, Tom Harper, once told me that if
you are a paramedic, you need to be cocky to survive. While I
never agreed with him completely, I understood that you need
the force of conviction to make your decisions, and you have to
be able to defend yourself. When I started as a paramedic, anytime a nurse or a doctor questioned me, I panicked and thought
maybe they were right and I was wrong. In time I learned to
trust myself.

The seventy-seven-year-old man in the nursing home has a
sudden onset of shortness of breath. He is sitting up, struggling
to breathe. His lungs sound like a dishwashing machine. His
skin is cool and sweaty, blue around the lips. His pulse is 132,
his blood pressure 200/120, his respiratory rate 46. He has a
history of emphysema and hypertension but none of congestive heart failure (CHF), which he is now suffering. In CHF the
heart's inability to pump efficiently causes the lungs to back up
with fluid, impeding the necessary exchange of fresh oxygen
into the bloodstream.

   The nursing home has him on an oxygen mask but at only
two liters. I hook the mask up to my portable oxygen and crank
it up to fifteen liters. We move the patient quickly out to the
ambulance, where I get an IV in his hand. I give him nitro-
glycerin under the tongue, and push 40 milligrams of Lasix
through the IV. The nitro will dilate his veins, causing fluid to
pool in his legs. The Lasix will cause fluid to move to his kid-
neys and soon cause him to urinate. The effects of these drugs
work to lessen the load on the severely overworked heart and

29

help clear the lungs so they can efficiently exchange oxygen into the bloodstream. I call the hospital on our radio and ask for a doctor. I describe the patient and ask for orders for an additional 80 milligrams of Lasix and 3 milligrams of morphine. The morphine, like the nitro, will dilate his veins and reduce the load on his heart. It will also help relax the man and take some of his anxiety away. He is still sucking away as we pull into the hospital. The medicine combo usually gets the job done, but it hasn't seemed to this time. I check the sheets; the man has yet to urinate, which ought to happen with that amount of Lasix.

They have a room ready for us. I give the report to a doctor and nurse. The nurse is dubious. "For my money, it's pneumonia or emphysema," she says, listening to the lungs. "I don't hear any rales. Just some wheezes." *Rales* are the bubbling sounds of fluid in the lungs.

"How much money do you have?" I say. "It's CHF."

"He has no history of CHF. I hear no rales, and he hasn't urinated," the nurse says. She lifts the sheets and pulls her hand back suddenly. The pee is streaming out of the man. For the first time, the patient looks relaxed. "I guess it could be the end of a CHF episode," the nurse concedes.

"Thank you," the patient says when I tell him they'll take good care of him. "Thank you."

What the hospital staff doesn't always understand is the patient we present them with is not always the same patient we saw when we walked into the room. Our interventions have made the difference.

I always want to be perfect; it's what people expect from medical professionals. However, like most everything in life, you never bat a thousand. You don't like to think that you can come up short.

It's three in the morning when I get sent to a wealthy neighborhood in West Hartford for a chest pain call. An attractive woman in her late forties lies on her bed and won't answer my questions. "Just take me to the hospital," she says. "I've never had pain like this before. My husband waited too long to call you."

I touch her forehead. It feels warm to me. Her color is good. Her pulse feels a little faint. My partner says he can't hear the blood pressure. I listen and get 96/60. Her husband says she had four martinis at dinner, which was unusual for her, and she has been vomiting. "You want her on a mask?" my partner says.

"A cannula will be okay," I say.

I put her on the monitor, thinking all along this is bull-shit. My three-in-the-morning stare sees a normal rhythm. I check all three leads—the same. I run an ECG strip and put it in my pocket.

"Where exactly is the pain?" I ask the woman.

"Just take me to the hospital," she says.

"I need you to help me here," I say.

"I'm not being a crybaby," she says. "Just take me there."

I feel the urge to snap at her, to call her a whiner.

My partner gets the stair chair and we carry her down. In the ambulance under the brighter light, she does look a little pale to me. I realize the light in the house and her makeup have fooled me. I feel her skin again. It feels a little cooler, but it is hard for me to tell because the night is cold and my hand is cold. We go on a priority two, and I put in an IV on the way. I don't give her a nitro or morphine because her blood pressure isn't quite high enough, plus I'm not buying this as cardiac. It's just some rich lady who had too many martinis.

In triage I tell the nurse, chest pain with vomiting. The woman had four martinis and it started after dinner. They send us down the hall. I feel her forehead again, and I can say it definitely feels cool. In the room, I give my report to the nurse.

"I'm not a crybaby," the woman says. "I've never felt pain like this before."

I label the blood tubes I drew, then go write my report. When I come back, the woman is vomiting again. There are two nurses and two doctors in the room. I hear one of them mention morphine. I see the twelve lead on the table and glance at it. Elevated T-waves, it says, have physician review. I ask the doctor who has just left the room what he thinks is going on. "She's having a heart attack," he says.

I walk back out to the car. I reach in my pocket and pull out the ECG strip, which I couldn't find when I was writing my report. I look at it now. There is a small but distinct elevation there. Elevated T-waves are an indication of a heart attack. I looked right at it but didn't see it. The three-in-the-morning stare. I missed it. I missed everything on that one. I swallow hard. You go for months thinking that you're doing a pretty good job, then boom, you blow one like this. I did some things right. I put her on the monitor. I gave $O_2$, though I should have gone with a higher concentration through a mask. I stair-chaired her, rather than making her walk. I put in an IV. I went on a priority. I got her to the hospital. What I didn't do was get enough sleep.

\* \* \*

On *Rescue 911*, every critical patient is saved. That's not real life. Sure we save some critical patients, but often if the body has betrayed its owner there is little we can do to reverse events. Being perfect, or close to it, doesn't matter.

The seventy-year-old woman was sitting in a chair when she collapsed and vomited. When we get there she is lying on the kitchen floor. She is alert and oriented but has no radial pulse, and I can't hear a blood pressure. Her stomach is large and mis-shapen. I touch below the belly button and can feel a pulsing mass. She denies that she is in any pain. She is just dizzy when she tries to get up. We get her on the stretcher right away and I say to Arthur, "Let's up-tempo this one."

In the ambulance, I say, "We're just going to use the lights and sirens to get through traffic, so don't you worry, okay?"

"Whatever you say," she says. "I don't suppose I am going to die, am I?"

"We're going to try not to let that happen. I'm going to give you an IV and run some fluid into you to get your blood pressure up a little bit."

I lay her arm on my knee, wrap a tourniquet around it, and look for the biggest vein I can find.

"I'm supposed to have surgery next week. I have an aneurysm in my stomach, I think," she says. "They took X rays yesterday at the medical office in West Hartford. Is that what made me pass out?"

"I think so. The aneurysm may be leaking."

"Oh, dear."

Triple A means an aortic abdominal aneurysm, where the wall of the descending aorta, the main blood vessel out of the heart to the lower extremities, bulges and thins. If it tears open, you exsanguinate. It can happen all at once, or it can slowly rip, the aortic wall stretching thinner and thinner like a balloon. In a dissecting aortic aneurysm, the blood gets into the wall of the vein and flows between the layers of the wall, producing a terrible tearing sensation. The elderly and those with high blood pressure are most susceptible to triple As. The only cure is surgical intervention to repair or replace the damaged aortic wall. In the field we treat a triple A like a trauma rather than a medical call. Load and go, oxygen, two large bore IVs, military antishock trouser (MAST) pants if you have time to put them on, and call the hospital and let them know what you are coming with so they can have a surgical team standing by.

"You are going to feel a little poke now," I say as I put a sixteen-gauge IV catheter in her arm. I get the flash, and advance it. She needs the biggest needle possible, but I was worried a fourteen gauge was too big for her vein. The sixteen just fit. I attach the IV bag. The fluid runs great. I just want to put in enough to reach a blood pressure of 90. The main thing is if her aneurysm bursts, I can let the fluid pour in, but if she bursts, there is little I can do to save her.

"You have such a nice knee," she says. "It's very comforting."

"Thank you. Do you have any pain in your back at all?"

"Just a little. It's nothing really."

I call ahead to the hospital, using the key words: "pulsing mass in the stomach," "tests that confirmed an aneurysm," "BP only 90, pulse weak."

At the hospital we wheel her right into room 14, where an attending physician is waiting to get a glimpse. The mass in her abdomen is huge. You can see it pulsing. The staff looks at each other. This may be too late. "That young man had such a nice knee," she says to the nurse. "Why are there so many people here?"

We're sent to West Hartford and find a naked man lying on the carpeted basement floor. He has some alcohol on his breath and is thrashing about. I try to get a blood pressure, but I can't keep him still. He vomits and I notice some black coffeelike grains, but then I look harder and see it is just spinach. We try to get him on the stretcher, but he can't sit still. "My back is killing me," he says. He violently scratches his back but gets no relief from it.

"Lie still," Arthur says, but he can't. We put him on the monitor and an $O_2$ mask, and strap him down tight, but he is screaming with pain. In the back of the ambulance, I put in a sixteen in one arm. We head out lights and sirens. I put in another sixteen on the way. He is thrashing so much he is now lying on the monitor. I try to ask him questions but he just swears at me. I can't hear a blood pressure. He keeps punching himself in the back, trying to get at the pain. I radio ahead. Unable to get pressure. Tearing sensation in back.

Neither patient makes it out of surgery alive.

*   *   *

Sometimes you get the job done and look like a hero, even when no one else knows how close you came to screwing up.

I get called for a man barely responsive, just got out of the hospital for a heart bypass. A police officer meets us at the curb. "He looks awful, cold clammy."

The man is slumped backward in a chair at the kitchen table. He is ashen white. His eyes look helpless, as if he is saying to me, *Just let me die.* He has massive fresh scars running the length of his inner thighs and down his chest, the surgical stitches still visible. He looks like a dead man risen from the grave, a ghost. I quickly feel his pulse. Very irregular. His wife hands me a long list of his medications on a tattered index card.

Mega heart meds. "He just had surgery. He has a terribly weak heart," the wife says.

"Let's just get him out of here," I say to Arthur. They want him to go to Hartford hospital, and we are a good fifteen minutes away. I put an oxygen mask on his face and turn it on full. We lift him up onto the stretcher. He is heavy, dead weight. I put him on the heart monitor and see three premature ventricular contractions (PVCs) right in a row. A bad sign. I am thinking this man may go into cardiac arrest before I can get him to the hospital. We hustle him outside and into the back of the ambulance. I tell my partner to head to Hartford on a priority. I'll do everything en route.

The man keeps looking at me, saying nothing. He seems dazed, as if life has knocked him down for the last time and what he is seeing now is the final part of the final reel. The credits are about ready to roll as the light grows dim.

I take his blood pressure. It is 180/90. High. That doesn't seem right to me. He should be low. I get a large-bore IV in his left arm. I set the needle on the bench to do a routine blood sugar when I get a chance. I look back at the monitor. He is still having PVCs but not at the rate he was. The oxygen seems to be helping. In my mind, I am running through what I will say in my report on the radio. I will call Hartford, and they will get room fourteen—the cardiac room—ready so that when I wheel the patient in, their doctors and nurses will descend upon him, hoping to avert imminent death.

I look at the man again and feel the wheels turning in my head. What am I missing? I get this feeling something is staring me in the face and I am not getting it. I glance back at the list of medications his wife gave me. Lasix, Lanoxin, Vasotec, HCTZ, ASA, isosorbide, Zyprex, Moban, Accupril, Sinemet, Zantac, diltiazem, glyburide. Glyburide. Glyburide. The man's a diabetic.

I pick up the needle I left on the bench and tap out a drop of blood onto a chemstrip. The reading comes back 0-20. Way low. I take a amp of D50 (dextrose) out of my drug box and inject it through the IV line. D50 is half sugar, half water. It can wake up an unresponsive diabetic in less than a minute. The sugar-thick fluid is carried in the bloodstream right up to the brain.

When we arrive at Hartford, the patient's wife bursts into triage, undoubtedly having braced herself for the possibility that her husband has expired en route to the hospital.

Instead he's sitting up on the stretcher with a big grin on his face. "Honey," he says. "This guy's the greatest paramedic in the world. He's got me all fixed up. Great fella."

She just starts crying and throws her arms around him, weeping huge grateful sobs.

"There, there," he says.

The triage nurse looks on at this inexplicable scene. Once the man woke up with the D50, I never bothered to radio the hospital. They only like reports for dire calls. "What do you have?" she asks.

"Diabetic," I say. "Gave him an amp of D50. He's doing much better." I fill her in on the rest of the details.

"Room fifteen," she says.

I imagine if I hadn't pieced it together until they discovered what I did—that his sugar was low—and the man woke up, healed, I would have felt like an idiot. Diabetic, huh? Oops.

Tunnel vision is a real problem. I got the heart bypass going in my head, the sight of the scars, the wife's comment about his bad heart, the PVCs on the monitor, all the heart meds. If I had been sent to an unknown or sent to a diabetic, I probably would have figured it out right on scene and revived him in the kitchen. At least I caught it in time.

# No Luck Left

We see a lot of bad accidents in this job and our share of truly injured people, but I am continually surprised at how lucky some people can be.

I'm working an overtime shift at night. My partner, Kristin Shea, and I are coming off the Sisson Avenue ramp when we notice an accident by the entrance divider. A car has spun into the guardrail. Several other cars are stopped. We tell dispatch we're going to stop and check for injuries. I see two people in the car. The one in the driver's seat seems okay. He is talking to the other passenger, who looks injured. The windshield is shattered. I go around to the passenger side. The hood is bent back and crashed through the windshield. The man's head is on the dashboard, pinned at the neck by the glass and the hood. He can't move it. I learn that the guy in the driver's seat is just another motorist—an off-duty firefighter who gets out of the car now and calls for the tactical unit on his radio. The guy with the wedged head is the driver. His feet are in the driver's seat. I can't believe what I am seeing. I go around and get in the driver's seat so I can talk to the guy whose head is facing me now. "Are you all right?"

"Yeah, I'm fine, I just can't move my head. Get me out of here, please."

He has alcohol on his breath, but he is alert. He has no other injuries. I inspect his head. He is wedged. The hood and glass are biting into his neck.

"You're lucky this didn't cut your head off," I say, then hold my tongue. He is not out of danger. One false move and that

37

glass could slice his jugular vein. I don't know how we're going to get him out. Leave it to the fire department. I can hear their sirens approaching.

Jeff Huffmire and Janice Mihalik in 471 show up on scene, and though we only have one patient, they stick around to help with the extrication.

Fire shows up and they conference repeatedly, trying to form a game plan. I have no idea what they will come up with. I'm glad it's not my decision. There is no margin for error.

"Just get me out of here, please," the guy says.

Janice sits on the other side, holding the guy's body up. We put a blanket over our heads to protect us from flying glass once the extrication starts. I try to slide a trauma dressing in between his neck and the glass, but the glass is right on the skin. Kristin gets the stretcher ready for quick extrication once we get him out and spikes a bag of fluid in the ambulance. Jeff stands close by the door to relay word to fire if anything starts to go wrong.

I hear a mechanical noise. I can't see what they are doing, but the extrication has begun.

The guy screams. "It hurts. It hurts. Stop! Stop!"

"Stop! Stop!" Janice and I yell. I picture his head dropping into my hands. Blood spurting from his severed neck.

They stop. There is a delay, while a new approach is decided upon.

"It's okay, you're going to be all right," I say.

"Just get me out of here, please," he says.

"You'll be okay," Janice says. "We'll get you out."

I hear more creaking and mechanical sounds. My hand is by his neck, ready to pull loose at the first leverage. I picture the glass coming up quickly, then suddenly falling down, taking my hand with it.

It seems like we're there for an hour.

"Just get me out," he says.

Suddenly there is a pop, and his head is loose.

"Grab his neck," I shout to Janice as I ease him free.

She holds his neck. I call for the board and, under the glare of the TV cameras, we quickly extricate him. Remarkably he is all right. He just has an abrasion on his neck, though I worry that with the compression he suffered, he may have swelling. He'll also need his spine X-rayed. I put in an IV en route just as a precaution. Janice rides along with me and patches to the hospital.

We describe the scene to the doctors and anyone who will listen. "Never seen anything like it," Jeff says. "His head was wedged on the dashboard. This close, and he's dead.

"The fire department saved your life," Jeff tells him. "They screw up and your head is off. Plop! Just like that. Decapitated. Just your neck spurting blood. The end. Dead."

The man is very contrite.

When I come back with my paperwork done, I wish him well, then ask, "So what are the lottery numbers for tomorrow?"

"I don't know. Three-eight-two."

"Three-eight-two. All right."

I buy a ticket on the way home. The following morning I'm back on my regular shift with Arthur. "Hey, check the lottery numbers for me," I say as he reads the paper. I tell him about the call and how I bought a ticket figuring to capitalize on the patient's luck.

"Sorry," Arthur says. "Four-zero-three. No luck left."

# Saving Lives

I think most of us became EMTs to save lives. To be heroes. Both Arthur and I have saved lives. People walk the earth because of our skills and actions: The woman in cardiac arrest shocked back to life. The pregnant girl in anaphalactic shock, her pressure dropping and airway closing, saved by a critical shot of epinephrine. The man in congestive heart failure, his lungs filled with fluid, his skin cold and clammy, his pressure and pulse through the roof, slammed with Lasix, nitro, and morphine and then intubated as his respirations dropped.

Getting a chance to truly save a life is rare in this job. Not an everyday occurrence. When we do get called for the big one— not breathing, can't wake up, crashed into a wall at eighty miles an hour, shot in the head—the person is often already dead, and despite our very best efforts, they are not coming back. Only a few calls involve true life and death where our actions in a few critical minutes make the difference between a living, walking, talking, loving, laughing human being, and the morgue that very day.

Rick Ortyl gets sent to a choking. The woman is blue, not breathing. No pulse. Using his laryngoscope and Magill forceps, he scoops macaroni and cheese out of her throat, then intubates her, starts a line, runs epinephrine and atropine in, and brings the woman's heart back. Before he leaves the hospital, she is awake and profusely thanking him. As he narrates, I wish I was called for that one, that I was the one there with the Magills in my hand, that I was the one saving the life, making the difference, winning the glory, justifying my own existence.

Ed Grant, Shirley Lessard, Tom Harper, Rick Scanlon, Shawn Kinkade, Joel Morris; they all have fresh stories of saves. I am jealous of their calls, their opportunity, their success.

It's been a while since I've had a true save. Months. First you need the call, the moment. Then you need to deliver, to perform.

# Bag and Drag

We're called for a motor vehicle accident and find a large man who looks to be in his late forties or early fifties slumped across the seat of a car with light front-end damage. He is unresponsive. His pupils are pinpoint, and he has been incontinent. Beside him on the seat is an empty bottle of amitriptyline, a tricyclic antidepressant. He wears a bracelet that says he is a diabetic. Since there is no damage to the steering column, windshield, or invasion into the compartment, and the front-end damage is minor, we take him right out of the car without C-spining him. This, I am thinking, is a medical problem, not the result of an accident.

In the ambulance, I take his blood pressure—it is 200/120. His pulse is 84. He is in a sinus rhythm on the monitor. I put him on a nonrebreather at full power and get an IV in his arm. I am thinking heroin overdose. I give him 1.2 milligrams of Narcan, then an additional .8 milligrams. No change. His blood sugar is around 80, so I try an amp of D50. Still nothing. I recheck his pupils and notice they have dilated somewhat, so maybe there was some opiate in there, maybe mixed with the tricyclics. I listen to his lungs again, which were clear, and now I hear rales, the wet bubbly sound of fluid flooding into the lungs. I look at the monitor, and see he is having ST elevations—a sign of ongoing injury to the heart. I tell Arthur to drive like hell to the hospital and reach for my med box to draw up some Lasix. This man's case is beyond my ability to solve. I glance back at his pupils. One has gone back to being constricted, while the other stays dilated. I think he has a bleed in his brain. He starts seizing. By now we are at the hospital. In the cardiac room he gets intubated, and the doctor gives him Valium, more Lasix. The twelve-lead ECG shows a possible heart attack. He is sent up for a CAT scan, which shows a massive bleed. Everything is going wrong. Later the doctor says he thinks it all started with the bleed, caused by the man's hypertension, while the trauma to the system caused him to go into pulmonary edema, and the strain caused the heart to infarct. The car accident and the tricyclics were red herrings.

The man lives, but is permanently incapacitated.

Not all calls can be figured out. The key for us is to follow a logical train of thought, develop a style, a routine so we don't forget anything in the midst of the chaos of the call.

We try to know when we can fix the problem there or when we have to bolt and run. "Stay and play" versus "Bag and drag."

A fifty-year-old man collapses of a heart attack four blocks from the hospital and goes into cardiac arrest. I will work that man where he fell because I have the equipment and tools to bring him back, and if he is going to be brought back, it is going to be here. He cannot afford the time it will take to get him in the back of the ambulance, drive four blocks, unload him, and wheel him down the hall to the cardiac room. He needs immediate defibrillation, intubation, an IV with medications. Once I have him stabilized—either back alive, tubed with a round of drugs in the line, or shocked into a flatline—then I can move him to the hospital. But if that same man were shot in the chest, I would put him on a backboard and fly (doing IVs and intubation en route) to the hospital trauma room, where they would rush to get him upstairs to a surgeon or operate on him right there, cracking his chest, trying to sew the hole in his heart.

There is a concept called "the golden hour of trauma" and a concept called "the golden ten minutes." The idea is a trauma victim has an hour to get definitive treatment at the hospital, and you never want to spend more than ten minutes on scene. Spend more than ten, and there is hell to pay. But they are both just concepts. Some patients have two hours, or two days, or the rest of their lives. Some don't have an hour. Some don't have twenty minutes, some don't have ten, some don't have sixty seconds. Spending ten minutes on scene for a guy who doesn't have it to spend is wrong.

Much of the controversy about the death of Princess Diana centered on the French EMS system, which took over an hour to get her to the hospital. In France, they work on the trauma patients on scene and in the stopped ambulance, rather than trying to race them to a trauma center, getting done what they can on the fly. Many U.S. experts thought Diana would have lived had she been rushed to the hospital and gotten definitive care in an operating room.

When you come into the trauma room, you want to have your patient intubated, two large bore IV lines running, neatly C-spined, clothes all cut off and exposed, every bullet hole bandaged. Unfortunately, there often isn't time for that, particularly when you are dealing with people shot within blocks of the hospital.

We're called for a shooting, possibly two victims. We arrive to find only one victim—a nineteen-year-old male shot twice in the torso. We learn later the guy who shot him, whom he shot in return, was taken to the hospital by private car. Our patient is badly hurt. He is perspiring, pale, short of breath. He looks blankly at me and says nothing. Death reaching in. We load him quickly onto a board and get him in the back of the ambulance. He needs a surgeon.

"Drive!" I shout to Arthur. "Drive."

And he does. Like the wind.

I try to get a quick blood pressure but can't. His pulse is fast, weak, and thready. I have time only to rip the young man's shirt open and listen to his lungs to see if he has a tension pneumothorax—a collapsed lung caused by a rapid buildup of air in the chest, pressing against a lung, collapsing it—which could kill him before we can get him to the operating room. I can drive a large needle into the chest to release the air, but I don't hear a tension. His lung sounds are equal on both sides, though very shallow. I get out the ambu-bag and start assisting his respirations. There is no time to intubate as we already are pulling into the hospital emergency entrance.

I come in with nothing, no tube, no line, no monitor, the guy on a backboard, no C-collar, only his chest exposed, bagging him with the ambu-bag, and mumble, "The guy's shot at least twice in the side—there—I couldn't get a pressure, pulse is weak and thready, I'd guess around a hundred and twenty." His breathing is shallow, labored. They look at me like I am incompetent. They don't see the clock on the wall of my imagination, the track and field million-dollar scoreboard that shows me breaking the tape to the trauma room door at 3:59 from arrival on scene. I go down the hallway, stripping my soaked gloves off my hands, my whole body drenched in sweat. I sit down and start my run form. Seven minutes later I look up and imagine my ambulance pulling in. I get out of the back with the same patient, backboarded, intubated, two large bore lines running, monitor attached, and oh yeah, CPR in progress. Good job, they tell me in the trauma room, you gave it your best. They look at their clock. Call the time. Patient pronounced.

Meanwhile upstairs in surgery, the surgeons have a live body to save. Our patient will live to walk out of the hospital, live to shoot, and likely, to be shot again another day. Saving lives can be complicated. You just have to try to do your job the best you can.

# Baby Code

My portable radio crackles, "Stonington . . . Baby not breathing."

I'm outside the Hartford Hospital Emergency Department. Arthur is in the back EMT room writing up the run form from our last call—a minor rush-hour motor vehicle accident up on

I-91 near the Jennings Road exit. I've just finished restocking the ambulance, putting a long board back in under the bench, finding some straps, making head rolls.

Stonington is just a couple minutes from the hospital.

"Did they send a basic to that call?" I ask Melody Voyer and Jerry Sneed, the crew of 461, who are bringing their stretcher in to pick up a transfer out. A basic is a car without a paramedic, just two basic-level EMTs, who don't carry heart monitors, breathing tubes, emergency medicines, IVs, and other advanced life-saving equipment.

"Yeah. Eight-five-six," Melody says.

Jerry says, "That's Pam Piseeka. She already did one pedi code this week."

There must not be any paramedic units available nearby. "Do me a favor. Art's in the back room. Go tell him we might be getting a call."

I open up the passenger door of my ambulance, 471, and pick up the mike to the company radio. "Four-seven-one, do you want us to take that Stonington call? We can clear."

"Yeah, four-seven-one, go. Eight-five-six, advise when you get there. I'm sending four-seven-one from Hartford."

"Four-seven-one responding."

I turn to go into the ER to get Arthur. A young paramedic student who has been waiting for 482 to come pick him up for the day, asks, "Do you mind if I come with you?"

"Hop right in back," I say.

Arthur comes out the automatic doors.

"Baby not breathing," I say.

"Where?"

"Stonington."

We head out, lights and sirens on.

As we pull out onto Retreat Avenue, I turn and say to the rider in back, "There's an orange box on the shelf under the monitor. That's the pedi box. Open it and take out the pedi ambu-bag, and get it set up."

"Four-seven-one," our dispatcher says, "It's confirmed, cardiac arrest."

"Copy. Tell them we're coming."

As we try to cross Maple Avenue, a man driving a blue Lincoln, talking on a cellular phone, blows right in front of us.

Arthur curses and pushes the air horn.

We're at a dead stop.

Cars ignore us. A Bronco whizzes by, oblivious to our whirling lights. A Taurus races past. Then a pickup.

Arthur guns the engine. We're across.

I wonder what lies ahead. Will the kid be inside or out? Will I find only the mother or a crowd of hundreds? Is the kid going to be freshly down or long dead? Either way, we'll go to the Connecticut Children's Medical Center (CCMC) next to Hartford Hospital. We haven't heard 856 put out yet. They must be coming from farther away.

We're on Stonington now. Ahead on the right in the parking lot is a fire engine and a group of people gathered around a police car. They are waving at us, shouting. Two men are doing CPR on the baby.

I call back to the rider, "Get the half board out, lay it on the stretcher." The half board is a short wooden board that we will lay the baby on; it will provide support for CPR compressions. I say to Arthur, "I'm going to grab the baby and we're going to bolt."

"Four-seven-one, eight-fifty-six, how you doing?" the dispatcher asks.

"Put us out in ten seconds," I say. As Arthur pulls to a halt, I jump out and run over to the car, my eyes locked on the baby.

"Where the fuck have you been!" a firefighter shouts at me.

"Jesus fucking Christ!" another one shouts. "We've been here for five minutes. Where have you guys been?"

"Tell me what happened," I say.

"His mother woke up and found him not breathing," the cop says.

"Don't fuck around. He's not breathing. Don't fuck around," the other firefighter shouts.

I pick the baby up and cradle it across my right arm, its head in my hand. I start toward the car. It has a wide, round head, no neck. It is a white-blue color and stiff. It feels just like a CPR infant mannequin. I walk fast. Everyone is yelling and screaming, crying. I do CPR with my fingers. I raise the baby's head up to my face and press my lips to its cold mouth and breathe in. You are not supposed to do mouth-to-mouth. There is danger of disease. You use the ambu-bag, but I don't have it— it's in the ambulance, and I couldn't give it air while walking this fast anyway, and everyone is yelling. I blow tiny breaths. The chest rises slightly. They are the coldest lips I have ever kissed.

I get in back, lay the baby on the board. A firefighter jumps in. I shout to Arthur to drive. Pam Piseeka arrives in the other car; she gets in and says she'll do compressions. She lies over the baby and works her fingers on its chest, a large woman over the little doll of the cold blue baby, beating her fingers, trying to change this world. The student has the ambu-bag. "Ventilate," I say. He doesn't have the mask attached. I root through the box for it but can't find it.

"It's on the floor," Pam says. I spot it by my large black boot, grab it, tear off the plastic, and attach it to the ambu-bag. I hand it back to the student and he starts ventilating. I attach the oxygen tubing on the ambu-bag to the oxygen spigot on the wall and turn it up to fifteen liters per minute.

I hear our dispatcher on the radio. "I'll notify CCMC for you."

We're off on a priority one, full lights and sirens.

I attach the heart monitor to the baby's chest, three tiny star-shaped electrodes, one over the right upper side, one the left upper, the last on the left lower.

I look at the monitor screen. Flatline.

I open the airway kit and grab a small plastic tube and a steel blade, which I attach to the laryngoscope. "Out of the way," I say.

"He's going to intubate," Pam says.

I ease the teeth apart, then stick the blade in the mouth, lifting up the tongue, and sweeping it aside. The bulb at the end of the blade illuminates the throat. I look for the tiny white vocal cords that should be hanging from the top of my view. I don't see them. I pull out. "Ventilate."

I wait thirty seconds and go in again. I look. Nothing. "Screw it. Ventilate."

Pam pounds away with her fingers, tiny compressions a half inch deep. The student ventilates steadily.

We're out at CCMC. The back door opens and Mike Lambert, a paramedic from another car, is there. I pass him a portable $O_2$ bottle, which he sets at the foot of the stretcher. I unhook the in-house oxygen and pass him the tubing, which he hooks up to the portable. Arthur pulls the stretcher out. We wheel it in. There is a large crowd of doctors, nurses, and staff waiting for us. We go straight into room one. "We don't know when the baby went out," I say. "The mother woke up and found it not breathing. Asystole in all three leads. Couldn't get a tube. It's pretty cold and stiff."

Doctors examine the baby. It's got lividity and rigor, meaning the muscles have stiffened and blood has pooled in the lower parts of the body after circulation ceased. They put it on their monitor. Flatline. They keep doing CPR while they decide what to do. The baby's dead. Long dead. We all know that. There is no point in doing anything, but they can't quite stop.

It is a baby.

I walk out. The firefighters are all standing there. "Is it going to be all right?"

"Hey, sorry we yelled at you. It's just that you're always there before us."

"No, that's all right. You guys did great. You had the baby right there for us. It was down too long, but if it had a chance, you would have done your part great."

"Sorry, we were just upset." I see some teary eyes. These big men in their turnout gear who brave fire and danger every day. I understand what they are feeling. They were there for the terrible part. The mother running out, holding her baby. My baby! My baby! My baby's not breathing! Then the waiting. Waiting for us to come. Where the hell are they? No motion in the baby. No life. Just the mother screaming. Their fingers going up and down on the baby's chest. Using their giant adult ambu-bag to try to get air into its lungs, only able to give tiny squeezes. No motion at all. Nothing they can do.

There are two company supervisors at the hospital now to see how everyone is doing. This is the fourth baby code our company has done in a week. "Fine," I say tersely. "The baby was dead."

I hear Pam say, "No, I'm not all right. Twice in a week."

In the call she had earlier with her regular partner, Shawn Kinkade, the baby was found with its head between the bars of its crib, not breathing, but freshly down. Shawn tubed it en route to the hospital and got a round of drugs down the tube. The staff at Mount Sinai worked on the baby for over an hour, but they couldn't bring it back.

When you have a bad call, what you want most of all is a second chance, to get back out there and win this time.

Pam walks around, shaking her head. I can see her arms and hands, opening up, tensing, closing, opening again.

I go out to the car and get a run form. I go back inside. The baby has been called—pronounced dead. A woman doctor is asking everyone how they are. The firefighters are still standing around. They look pale, distraught.

I sit in the alcove to write my report. I look at the blank spaces. *Name.* I don't know it. *Sex.* I sit there stunned. I don't even know if it was a boy or a girl.

"I know we're all tough guys," Bill Terri-Savage, a supervisor, says to me, "but we're going to set up a CISD debriefing for anyone who wants it." CISD is critical incident stress debriefing, where everyone sits around and tells how they feel about the bad call they just went through.

"Fine," I say, looking straight ahead. "I'm okay."

"Just if you need it."

I nod.

I get up, get the name from a nurse, and write it down on my pad. It is a girl, four and a half months old. The mother is in the room, holding the baby in her arms, cradling her, rocking her. I go back and sit down in the alcove. I write my report:

4½-month-old female found not breathing by mom. Unknown down time. On our arrival HFD and HPD on scene. CPR in progress. Baby pulseless, apneic, cyanotic. CPR continued, compressions and ventilations. Transported priority one to CCMC. Asystole on monitor. Intubation attempted. No cords visualized. CPR continued. On arrival Pt still pulseless, apneic. Turned over to CCMC staff with full report.

I call for our times. *Dispatch and Respond:* 8:09. *Arrival:* 8:12. *Transport:* 8:14. *Destination:* 8:17.

The dispatcher asks how we all are. "The baby was dead," I say. "It looked like a CPR mannequin."

There is still a crowd in the ER. Arthur is standing by the nurses' desk, looking in at the mother holding her baby. He's got four kids of his own, all grown now and out of the house.

I think I want to be anywhere but here. "Let's go," I say to Arthur. "Let's get out of here. Let's go do some calls."

In the car, he sits behind the wheel for a moment before starting up the engine. "It's a shame," he says.

He's been on the job in this city seven years. He's been at EMS in one form or another—firefighter or EMT—for more than twenty-five. This is my third year in Hartford, eighth in EMS. We've been partners for almost a year, doing more than a thousand calls together. Shootings, heart attacks, strokes, diabetic shocks, assaults, burns, car accidents, drug overdoses, cut fingers, colds and flu, drunks. Most you forget about as soon as they are over. Others you carry with you.

A couple hours later, we're sitting outside Saint Francis. It's been quiet. We still haven't done another call. "Four-seven-one," the dispatcher asks us. "Are you interested in attending the CISD?"

Arthur looks at me.

"No," I say quickly. "I'm all right."

He says nothing.

"The baby was dead," I say. "There was nothing we could do. Unless you want to go. I'll leave it up to you."

He is a strong man. I kid him about all the ibuprofen he takes, but the two of us have carried huge patients up and down stairs by ourselves. We pride ourselves on never having to ask for a lift assist. But now for the first time I notice the gray in his mustache, the lines etched in his face. He looks as old as I've ever seen him.

"No, thank you," Arthur says back to the radio, his voice tired. "We're doing okay."

He puts the mike down, then takes off his glasses and pretends to rub a spot in them.

"I just want to do some calls," I say, determined. "I like to do calls."

I catch a small glisten in his eyes as he puts the glasses back on.

"I know you do," he says.

# STORY OF A LIFE

*I never want to lose my focus on the patient, on the person.*

# Respect

I never miss work and I am never late. I try to do my job well but the truth is there are some days I don't want to be here, days when I hate my job. When I find myself not caring. When I get testy, tired, snapping at patients—something that happens far more often than it should. I know that burnout is an occupational hazard. Burnout from too much stress. Burnout from lack of respect. Burnout from frustration. Burnout from finding out that what you love is not always what you want it to be. I see it in others, even in medics I respect, medics I revere. I guard against it in myself. I try to squash it down when it rears its head.

I want to be good, not just in the big bad ones, but every day, day in, day out. I want to treat everyone with respect. With care. Patient to patient. Heart attack to broken ankle. Migraine headache to massive stroke. My job is my church. Though I often fall short, every day I try to seek grace.

I want to allay my patients' fears, make them feel less alone. The fifty-three-year-old man who passed out on the treadmill and still feels a little shaky. The seventy-five-year-old stroke victim who can only squeeze my hand with her right hand, and though she tries, cannot speak. The twenty-five-year-old with asthma, who now on her second Ventolin breathing treatment, is finally starting to calm down. The eighty-three-year-old woman who has a fever and has been vomiting all night. I introduce myself. "My name is Peter. I'm a paramedic. How are you doing?" I try to listen to their stories, hear their complaints, their troubles. I tell them what I am doing for them. What they can expect. I lay my hands on them. My words are

55

soft. I try to look them in the eyes. When we get to the hospital and get them in their room, I introduce them to the nurse. I pass over care. I always try to touch their shoulder and say, "They'll take good care of you here."

I want to feel that what I do matters to someone, even if only for a moment.

# Life on Mars

We get called for an unresponsive diabetic on Brookfield Street. We're coming from Saint Francis, so it's taking us awhile. The dispatcher radios back asking for our ETA—the man is still unresponsive, she says.

"Put us out," I say, as Arthur pulls to a stop in front of the house.

The address is across the street from the Charter Oak Rice Heights Housing complex, World War II public housing. Once a model of its kind, it is now drug-ridden, litter-strewn, and targeted for demolition.

Two women in their sixties meet us at the door. "He's a diabetic," she says. "I can't get him up. My sister and I just got back from a trip to Massachusetts. I don't know how long he's been like this. He doesn't take care of himself."

The man is slumped in a chair in front of the TV, newspapers scattered on the floor, an empty ice cream carton and several bottles of beer on the table next to him. His skin has a blue hue. He is cold and very diaphoretic. His tongue is partially blocking his airway, producing a snoring sound when he breathes.

"When did you last see him?" I ask as I reposition his head so he can breathe easier.

"Two days ago," she says, "when we left on our trip. I knew I shouldn't have left him. He just doesn't care anymore."

I strap a tourniquet on his arm. It is a pretty good bet that he is hypoglycemic, meaning his blood sugar level is too low to sustain normal brain activity. Untreated, it can cause coma, then death. My worry is that he's been out so long he has already irreparably damaged his brain. I get the IV and hand Arthur the needle to do a chemstrip check, while he hands me the IV line.

He puts a drop of blood on the strip and a minute later wipes it off. "I'm not getting a reading," he says. "Too low to measure."

I already have the dextrose out. As I push the drug in, the man slowly starts to move, then opens his eyes, and looks around like Rip van Winkle. "Ah, Christ," he says.

"How are you?" I ask.

"George, I can't leave you alone," his wife says. "I called and you didn't answer. We had to come back."

"Maybe you should have left me," he says.

"What time do you remember last being up?" I ask.

"I don't know. I was watching TV, having a beer."

"He won't take care of himself," she says. "He thinks nothing about eating a quart of ice cream. He's going to kill himself."

The man grunts and shakes his head. "You came home too early," he says.

"I don't know what I'm going to do."

"We need to take you to the hospital," I say.

"Can't you just leave me here?"

"No, what I gave you won't last. You should get checked out, and they'll get you something to eat there." I am also thinking maybe they need to give him some counseling. "Maybe they can alter your medications."

He nods. He knows the routine.

We get him on the stretcher and out to the ambulance. Across the street, they have a fence up over a portion of the complex. A bulldozer is knocking down a two-story building. In a dwelling not yet targeted, a group of people sit out drinking beers while kids play in the dirt. They watch us take the man out on the stretcher and lift him into the back of the ambulance.

"So when do you think you were last alert?"

He shrugs. "I don't know. They should have just left me alone."

"You a baseball fan?"

"Detroit Tigers," he says, some life coming back in his voice.

"What place were they in when you last checked?"

He snorts. "Last," he says.

"Well, good news," I say. "They won the pennant. Al Kaline came out of retirement to lead them. The World Series starts today."

He laughs. "Get out of here," he says.

"Did you hear about California?"

"No."

"It fell into the sea."

"No, get out of here."

"I'm just trying to find out how long you've been sleeping. Hey, did you hear, they discovered life on Mars?"

"Yeah, I know, I saw that on TV," he says, "and it's a load of bull."

I laugh. "Who would have thought," I say. At least he was alert then.

"Life on Mars," he says. "I should live so long." He shakes his head.

"What was it—just some bacteria they found?"

"Bacteria," he says. "Life is people—Martians, spacemen—not germs, for God's sake."

"I hear you," I say.

We're stopped in the middle of the road, just down the street from his house, as a dump truck swings around and tries to back into the demolition site, its backup alarm beeping.

"There goes the neighborhood, huh?" I say.

"Forty years I've lived here," he says. "I worked for an insurance company. I had the money to move anytime. My wife wanted me to move years ago when it first started going downhill, but I like living here. It's my house. I raised my family here. That counts for something."

"I'm sure it does."

He shakes his head. "Call me stubborn," he says. "I like drinking beer, eating ice cream. How else am I supposed to live?"

"I don't know."

"They came back too early," he says.


# Lord Randal


"There he is on the corner," I say from two blocks off.

"It's Randal," Arthur says. "Joan and I picked him up yesterday."

Randal Martinez is a regular. I've picked him up myself seven or eight times. Hardly a day goes by that we don't see him in the tube station at Hartford or in the crisis unit at Saint Francis. He's a strongly built man in his late forties. He drinks till he can't stand up, then he sits down on the sidewalk and waits for someone to come get him. He's never so out of it that we have to use ammonia inhalants to wake him up or transport him comatose.

We park, get out, and stand over him, putting on our latex gloves as we greet him.

"Hey, hey, let me ask you," he says. "I think I killed somebody."

"You killed somebody!" I say in a loud voice.

"Shh, shh, shh," he says, smiling.

"You sure you want to be telling us that?" Art says.

"I stabbed her," he says.

*"You stabbed her!"* I shout.

"Shh, shh, shh," he says.

"Okay, okay," I say in a whisper. "You stabbed her?"

"No, I shot her," he says.

*"You shot her!"* I shout.

He holds his finger up to his mouth.

"Okay, okay," I say in a whisper. "You shot her. *Where's the dead body?"*

He starts laughing and motions me to be quiet. "No, no, no, she OD'd."

"OD'd?"

"No, no, no, I'm just kidding. I was just wondering what you guys would do if I really did."

"We'd take care of you. We'd raise her from the dead. We wouldn't let you take a murder rap."

"You're my friends."

"What hospital do you want to go to?"

"ADRC."

"You're sure you're not on the banned list?"

"Give it a try?"

"He needs his Tegretol levels checked," Arthur says. "It's what they said yesterday."

"Howabout we take you to Saint Francis?"

He nods and offers us his hands to help lift him. We get him to his feet. He is slightly unsteady. With each of us holding an arm, we walk him toward the ambulance.

"Jeez, Randal," Arthur says, "you must cost us one hundred thousand dollars a year easily."

"Hey, hey, don't say that about me."

"You don't have to pay it. The taxpayers have to foot the bill."

Randal drops his arms down and makes fists.

"Easy, easy," I say.

"I don't like him talking about me like that. I'm a veteran."

"I didn't mean it personally," Arthur says.

"I fought for this country. Eighteen-year-old Puerto Rican. I seen my best friend killed. Don't talk to me. I cost you?"

"I'm sorry," Arthur says.

Randal spits on the floor. "Fuck you for saying that."

Arthur laughs and hold his hands up. "I didn't mean anything." He bows. "I am not worthy. I am not worthy."

"Come on, Randal," I say.

He is too unsteady and unpredictable to step up into the back of the ambulance, so I pull the stretcher out, and we get him on it.

"Did you fight in the war?" he asks Arthur.

"No," Arthur says. "I didn't get drafted."

"How 'bout you?" Randal says to me.

"He wasn't old enough," Arthur says. "He's just a baby."

We get him in the back. Randal is still angry at Arthur. I tell Arthur to just head to Saint Francis.

"How old are you?" Randal asks me.

"Forty," I say. "I was fourteen when the war ended."

"Good, you're lucky. How could he say that about me? Costing him money. It cost me. Hey, what's your name? I forget."

"Peter," I say.

"Peter, Peter, pumpkin eater . . ."

I join him. "Had a wife and couldn't keep her, / put her in a pumpkin shell / and there he kept her very well."

He laughs. "I like rhymes and poetry."

"You like poetry? I've got a poem for you." I have been listening to a tape of great poetry. This poem caught my fancy and I have been memorizing it. I put on a thick Irish brogue and lean toward him. " 'Oh where ha'e you been, Lord Randall, my son? / O where ha'e you been, my handsome young man?' "

"Randal. That's my name."

I hold my finger to my lips. " 'I ha'e been to the wild wood: mother, make my bed soon, / For I'm weary wi' hunting, and I fain would lie down.' "

His eyes are fixed on me. I press on. " 'Where got you your dinner, Lord Randall my son? / Where got you your dinner, my handsome young man?' / 'I dined wi' my true love: mother, make my bed soon, / For I'm weary wi' hunting and I fain would lie down.' "

I hear Arthur laughing in the front. I have Randal's rapt attention. "What got ye to your dinner, Lord Randall my

son? / What got ye to your dinner, my handsome young man?' /
'I got eels boiled in bro': mother, make my bed soon, / For I'm
weary wi' hunting and I fain would lie down.' / 'What became
of your bloodhounds, Lord Randall my son? / What became of
your bloodhounds, my handsome young man?' "

I hesitate a moment, an ominous mood shift. " 'O they
swelled and they died: mother, make my bed soon, / For I'm
weary wi' hunting, and I fain would lie down.' "

"They died?" he says.

" 'O I fear ye are poisoned, Lord Randall my son! / O I fear
ye are poisoned, my handsome young man!' "

I hold my hand to my chest. "Oh yes, I am poisoned: mother,
make my bed soon, / for I'm sick at the heart, and I fain would
lie down.' "

"That's good," he says. "I like that. Poetry."

"It's called 'Lord Randall,' " I say.

"They wrote that about me, huh?"

"Or maybe some other Randal like you."

"Let me tell you one. It's not really a poem, but I am going to
tell it anyway."

"All right."

"It's more like a story about what happened to me."

"Okay."

He motions me closer, but the alcohol on his breath causes
me to pull back a little.

"It's a funny little world," he says in a soft voice, his eyes
looking right into mine. "Sometimes, you just want to draw a
big question mark, and say why."

"I guess."

"Eighteen years old, I'm lying in some country I never heard
of before. I'm just a Puerto Rican. I don't know why I'm there."
He shrugs. "But it doesn't matter. No matter what I think, I'm
still there. Can't do nothing about it. My friend, lying next me.
I'm a medic, but I can't do anything."

I nod.

"When I came back to Brooklyn, it was raining. I went to my
house, and my wife, she was in bed with a man." He pauses.
His eyes are looking back into his mind, then he focuses back

on me. "I threw them both out into the rain. The guy had three hundred sixty-five dollars." He pats his side. "I pocketed it. He said, 'I want my clothes.' I said, 'No, but you take her with you.'"

"That was telling him."

"Take her with you." He nods. "I was a hell-burner. My friends came to me and said, what'd you want to do about it? I said nothing."

"What happened?"

"They killed them."

"They killed them?"

"They killed them."

"You're kidding. Both of them?"

"I was a hell-burner. Eighteen years old."

"That's some story."

"It was raining," he says.

We're at the hospital. Arthur opens the back door and we pull the stretcher out.

"Hey, Randal," the security guard says. "Back again."

"Hey, man, how are you?"

In triage, we put him in a wheelchair. Arthur takes him to the back while I write up the run form. When I finish, I see them walking back down the hall. "He didn't want to be strapped down," Arthur says.

"Fuck that," Randal says. "I don't need the straps today." He looks up at me. "You're a big guy. You play basketball?"

"I used to," I say. "Not much anymore."

He edges in close to me. "Put your arms up like you're going for a rebound." When I do, he pokes an elbow at my belly. "I could clear you out under the boards."

"You probably could. You're a hell-burner."

"Hey, how'd you know that?"

"I know a lot of things."

He laughs and nods, then says, "See you later, man."

We watch him walk out—stumble out—the ER door.

"Scumbag," Arthur says.

I say nothing. I just watch him make his way down the street. The afternoon is cloudy and overcast.

# What About the Man?

We're taking a forty-year-old woman with body aches to the hospital on a priority three, no lights, no sirens. I'm driving, talking to her companion, the man who called 911.

"But she says she ain't feeling right," he says, "and I don't want to mess around with that, you hear what I'm saying? She's just an acquaintance, but she got a heart murmur. Is that bad? I know she had a few cocktails, but I said, honey, we going to take you to the hospital. Can't mess around with that. My friend died last week. Gone from the world. He's a diabetic, got so bad, he lost his bowels. We drive together. He said he want to carry his load. I said you can't be driving shitting all over the place, messing up, long drive, you going to the hospital. I took him. He went into a coma, and now he's gone. I told the boss, and the first thing he say, 'How's my load?' How's my load! He asking about the load. What about the man! You hear what I'm saying?"

"Yes, I do," I say.

"What about the man? Work for him making him money all these years, and he asks about the load. What about the man? What this world coming to? He trained me, that man, I known him twenty years. Hardworking man. You hear about those three people shot? Man walks into another man's house he don't even know, shoots three people over drugs. What the world coming to? Right in front of his kids. People dying. Friends dying. Damn. I'm a hardworking man myself. I can't understand it. You hear what I'm saying?"

I nod. "Yes, sir, I do. You've got a point."

"I know I had a few cocktails, but I don't get much chance.

**64**

I'm working all the time. I'm a truck driver, hauling those loads, can't be drinking with those eighteen-wheelers cutting in front of you, can't be drinking when you carrying a load, you know what I'm saying. I hope she all right. She got a heart murmur. I know both of us had some cocktails. I hope she all right. You can't mess around with someone's life, you hear what I'm saying?"

"I do," I say. I do.

# An Old Man, a Crack Girl, and a Rat

We're called to an unknown on Albany Avenue. It is seven-fifteen on a cold, rainy morning. The address is an old private home. There is a weathered FOR SALE sign out front; the paint is chipped and faded. We're on the sidewalk looking up the cracked stone steps at the house, which looks abandoned. I'm thinking maybe this is another heroin OD. I've done them up and down this block.

"You in the right place." A woman wearing a green snow jacket and eating a sticky bun walks past us. "Up here."

We follow her through the door, which she opens without a key. The odor hits us before we are in the house. Garbage. Urine. The house is dim and looks ransacked.

"He in here," she says, leading us into a back bedroom that is pitch-black.

I hit the wall switch, but nothing comes on. There is no bulb in the ceiling fixture. "Do you have a light that works?"

"No," she says, "He there on the floor."

In the darkness I can see the shape of a man, lying on his back. I grab his shoulder and give it a rub. He is breathing. "How old is he?"

"I don't know. He can't walk."

"Why?"

"'Cause I already tried to get him up."

I shine a penlight in his face. He is probably in his seventies or eighties, strongly built. I feel a hand grab my leg. I am thinking maybe a stroke.

"Let's just get him out of here," I say to Arthur. "Get him in the front room where we can see what's going on."

We lift him up. He has only one leg, and no balance.

"Maybe diabetic," Art says.

"Good thought."

He grabs us hard with his arms, fighting us, but we lug him into the front room and set him on the couch.

"What kind of medical problems does he have?" I ask the woman.

"I don't know."

"Do you know what medications he takes?"

"No."

She is probably in her middle thirties, but is watching us with all the fascination of a five-year-old as she chews her cinnamon bun, the sticky goo collecting on her lips and face.

"Who are you?"

"I just look after him."

He is battling with us, his eyes open, but doesn't speak. He is strong for an old man. Arthur is holding him down so I can get an IV in. I sit on his arm and stick him and get a flashback, but suddenly he gets his arm loose and knocks me off balance. His head flies back and hits the wall behind the couch. It stuns him for a moment. The needle falls to the floor. Just as I reach for it, something furry runs across my boot. "Jesus Christ! Did you see that?"

"A mouse," Arthur says.

"A mouse! It was a fucking rat. Hold him down for me."

We get back on him, Arthur pinning his shoulders, me sitting on his arm again. Instead of going for a smaller gauge, I go for one bigger. I take a sixteen out of my shirt pocket and jab it hard through his tough skin at the vein that runs along his wrist. I'm in. I draw off four tubes of blood, screw on the IV line Arthur has spiked for me, and tape it down. Only then do I get off the patient's arm.

Art checks the blood sugar on our glucometer.

"He got one of those machines, too," the woman says.

"Are you related to him or are you his girlfriend or something?"

"No, I just stay here."

"Blood sugar thirty-nine," Arthur says.

"Well, there you have it." His sugar should be up above eighty, at least. The brain needs sugar to function.

Arthur hands me an amp of D50 from the bag. I push it through the line into his vein. He starts to come around.

He looks at me, puzzled. "Did you hit me?"

"No, you banged your head against the wall."

He looks about the room. His eyes focus on the woman. "Is that Mary? Hah. It is. Look at her eating."

"Your blood sugar was low," I say. "We just gave you some sugar right into your veins. Now we have to take you to the hospital."

"I go to the VA."

"If Saint Francis is all right, we'll take you there."

"That's okay." He looks back at the woman. "You always eating. Look at her. That's my girl. Always eating my food."

"Put your leg on and go to the hospital," she says.

"Mary, Mary, Mary," he says. Then to us, "She wants me out of here, so she can have a party. Bring all her friends."

We help him get his leg on and get dressed.

"You got your money?" she says.

He reaches under the cushion and takes out three crumpled dollar bills, which he sticks in his pocket.

"You got your hat?"

He looks around and finds it on the floor on top of some loose newspapers.

With his hat, overcoat, and cane, he looks distinguished. We walk him slowly down the steep stairs.

"Don't let all the heat out," he calls back to Mary, who stands in the doorway.

"You go to the hospital," she says.

\* \* \*

In the back of the ambulance, I ask him where he was in the service.

He smiles. "Okinawa, Iwo Jima, Saipan."

"Iwo Jima," I say, impressed. "Were you one of the guys who raised the flag, who held it high?"

"Marine Corps. *Semper fi.*"

"So who's this Mary?"

He laughs. "Mary? She's a street girl. She's out all night looking for crack."

"She lives with you?"

"When she's not out looking for crack."

"So what's her relation to you?"

"There's no relation. I met her at McDonald's about a year and a half ago. She followed me home. Next thing I know she was living there. She's got a room and bed. She eats all my food."

"You don't sleep with her or anything do you? She's not your girlfriend?"

"I wouldn't put it in there. You don't know what's been in there."

"A man has to have standards."

"She's no good. She just wants me out of the house, bring her crack friends over. Have a party."

"Why don't you toss her out?"

"She said I send her back out on the street, she'll break all the windows in my house. When she gets too wise with me, though, I put her in the death hold."

"The death hold?"

"The two of us have an understanding."

"She looks after you."

"Eats all my food."

"Well, she did you a service today."

He laughs. "She's just out for herself."

After the call, Arthur and I talk about the old man and the woman. I wonder whether or not her living off him constitutes elder abuse and whether we ought to report anything to the authorities. The guy is pretty much at her mercy. His sister lives in a nursing home. His wife is dead. But she did call 911, after all.

"I get the sense he likes having her around," Arthur says.

"Yeah, me too."

A month later we get called for an unconscious man, police and fire on the scene. "We were here before, weren't we?" Arthur asks as we walk up the steps, carrying our gear. "What was it for?"

"It was the diabetic."

"I don't remember."

"Sure you do. Remember that guy and the crack girl?"

"Yeah, yeah, that's right."

A fireman meets us at the door. "I don't know if they told you. He's been here awhile."

"Oh, okay, no they didn't." He leads us into the room, and there the man is on the couch, lying on his side, one arm dangling down to the floor. He is dead, cold, and stiff. Long gone. Days.

"Look out, there's a rat around here," the fireman says.

"I remember him," I say.

"That's right," Art says. "We've been here before."

We attach our monitor. I put one lead on each wrist, the third on his left side. I run the six second strip. Flatline.

"The hero of Saipan, Okinawa, and Iwo Jima."

"At least he died at home," Art says.

I unhook the monitor. "Beats a nursing home." I rewind the cable chord.

A cop comes in. He is trying to find out who the guy is.

We tell him his name. His sister lives in a convalescent home. There's a crackhead named Mary who lives here.

The cop nods. "Yeah, we know her. No one has seen her for a week."

"That explains this," I say to Art.

"No one to call for help."

Then I look down at his hand on the floor. "Look at this," I say. I shine my light on his fingers. The meat of one fingertip has been eaten down to the bone. Another chunk of flesh is gone from his thumb. He has been nibbled on by the rat.

"There you have it," I say. "End of story."

# Story of a Life

Sometimes at the health club, my feet whirling around on the exercise bike have slowly come to a stop, and I have gotten off the bike and walked out in the middle of a workout, tired, discouraged, beaten. I go home and sit on the couch. I look at the paper without reading it. I watch TV. Hours pass. I wonder what's wrong with me. Where's my motivation? Where's my energy? I've struggled against this fatigue almost all my life. I think how when I was a little boy walking to the store with my mother, sometimes I would get tired and just stop and squat and refuse to go on. But then she would either pick me up or more likely grab me by the arm and yank me along. Today life is sort of like my mother. I can sit for a little while, but life swoops me back up and pulls me along till I gain my feet and keep going on my own. I do get in funks and get depressed, but I've never been to the point of just plain not going on.

I'm working with Pam Duguay. She is a tall, athletic twenty-six-year-old who is going to paramedic school. I like working with her because she is enthusiastic and wants to learn. We're out in an exclusive neighborhood in West Hartford on a chest pain call. We've been there with a cop for ten minutes, trying to get into the locked house. The cop says the dispatcher has the man on the phone, but the code he's gotten for the garage door doesn't work.

I think he's probably on the floor, having the big one, one

hand clutched to his chest, the other holding the phone, as he gasps out the numbers to the garage door, barely able to say the words to the nervous dispatcher.

The cop breaks a windowpane in the garage, unclasps the window lock, and lifts it up. I lay a towel over the broken glass and climb into the garage over a large bag of peat moss. I check the door leading into the house. It is unlocked. I run up the stairs, then up to the second floor, where I enter the spacious bedroom.

A man in his sixties sits in a king-size bed, covers pulled up to his waist, the night table light on. The TV plays *Good Morning America*. "Are you okay?" I ask.

"No, I'm not well," he says.

His face is flushed—he doesn't look too bad. I touch his forehead. He feels a little sweaty.

"What's going on?"

"I can't get up."

"Are you having any chest pain or discomfort?"

He shakes his head.

I have him squeeze my hands and wiggle his feet, which he does without a problem.

"I was in the bathroom shaving," he says, "and I felt weak, so I got back in bed and was afraid to get up. Maybe I can get up now."

I excuse myself for a moment and go downstairs and open the front door for Pam and the cop. "He's okay," I say. "I think we're dealing with a psych case."

Back upstairs, we give him a full checkup. Aside from his blood pressure being a little high, physically he seems okay. We agree to take him to Hartford Hospital to get checked out. "I know it may be a waste of time, but I'll feel better about it. I'm just afraid of going out, afraid something will happen to me." He starts to sob.

Pam pats his shoulder. "It's all right. You'll be okay."

The cop shakes his head and walks out of the room.

Twenty minutes later, we are finally leaving the house with the patient. I carry his suitcase, which he has spent twenty minutes packing: walking about his room, getting his slippers and green bathrobe out of the closet, two pressed white shirts from the bureau, along with socks and underclothes, and his shaving kit.

"It's not a good idea to take all this stuff to the ER," I tell him. "It may get lost. In all likelihood, you'll be back home later today."

"I know, I just want to be prepared," he says. "I'll keep it with me."

Pam and I roll our eyes. Downstairs, he takes the morning paper from the breakfast table and stuffs it into the suitcase.

We finally get on our way, no lights, no sirens.

"This ever happen to you before?"

"I've just not been feeling great lately."

"What do you do for a living?"

"I own my own business."

"That's good."

I don't ask him much else. As I write my run form, I think this is a good story to tell. We get called for a chest pain, have to break into the guy's house and climb over the fertilizer, and he ends up spending twenty minutes packing his suitcase. You meet all kinds.

I've been doing a lot of interesting calls lately. To me a call is interesting if it is medically challenging or if I see something in the people or the situation that makes me think about life and the human race in general. I got sent to Hartford Hospital to take a young woman to the McLean home in Simsbury, where my mother spent the last years of her life before succumbing to multiple sclerosis. This thirty-year-old woman's problem is a sudden malevolent cancer that has overwhelmed her body in just a few months' time. A troubling headache led to shoulder pain, to stomachaches, to a doctor telling her her condition was terminal. She is constantly nauseated, can barely even tolerate sipping water, feels pain despite the morphine pumped continually into her body. She is going to McLean to die. I tell her it's a very nice place, and she seems interested in this. I don't tell her my mother died there, just that it is one of the nicest facilities in the state. I am impressed that this seems

to please her. I think if I were her, I wouldn't care about anything. How do you face dying? I read her name on the obituary
page before the week is out.

Arthur and I get sent to a shooting off Albany Avenue. We
climb up a narrow staircase in an abandoned house to find a
man lying on the floor, holding his bloody groin, where a
close-range shotgun blast has left a gory mess. "Is it going to
work? Can they make it work?" he moans as we race him to the
trauma room. I try not to look the bloody crater lake where his
manhood used to be. At the scene, the cop asked him if the
shooting was over drugs. He shook his head and moaned. Later
that night, while the surgeons work to put his penis back on, a
woman comes in with a thumb missing and powder burns on
her hand. Seems that in her rage at him, she held her hand a
little too close over the edge of the sawed-off gun. Change
comes quickly. One moment there, the next gone.

Our company is being sold to a large national medical transportation company, so everyone is a little on edge. Change,
which can be good, is also unsettling. People are worried about
their jobs. Our union president tells us we have nothing to
worry about, but that doesn't help much. I believe our jobs are
safe. What worries me is the working conditions. Now I arrive
in the morning, check out my ambulance, get on the road, do
the calls, and no one bothers me. I worry we will have to wear
new uniforms with ties that make us look like fast-food man-
agers, and supervisors will write us up if our shoes aren't
shined. Every time it gets slow and I stretch out in the back of
the ambulance, a supervisor will knock on the back window,
chew me out, write me up. They will change my schedule to
Monday through Friday nine-to-five. They will make me shave
my mustache, trim my hair. Maybe they'll take a dislike to me,
and then I will get fired. It's a scary thing to lose control. I am
in many ways in my prime. I am healthy, strong. I love what I
do, but in this job you see the arbitrariness of life, how brutal it
can be. You try to think it can't happen to you, but you know

any day, month, year, your number could come up. It's a matter of when, not if.

A week goes by and it's the next Thursday and Pam is working with me again. She tells me about the restaurant her boyfriend took her to and the movie they saw afterward. Her boyfriend is a new medic, a nice twenty-two-year-old kid. She talks about him in a way I wish a girlfriend talked about me, with a sort of openness about the future and belief in good things to come. If he wants to go to California, she says, that'd be great. We're young, we can try it out. I think if he doesn't ask her to marry him soon, he is a major knucklehead, though I have to admit, at twenty-two I wouldn't have been able to recognize the traits I see in her now. At twenty-two, I wanted a thousand women. At forty, I sometimes think about the women in my past who I let slip by the wayside. As she tells me about the cruise she and her boyfriend are planning to take this summer, I feel some regret about my old college sweetheart and how we should have gone on more vacations together. I remember one we did go on, after we had already decided to break up. We went to New Hampshire to climb Mount Washington. It took us five hours to get to the top, and she wanted to stop several times along the way, but I kept us going. Can't quit, can't quit. I knew as long as we kept moving we'd get there. When we finally did get to the mountaintop, we were both thrilled. She was so glad I had kept us moving all the way to the summit. I had brought a small bottle of champagne, and we drank it out of plastic glasses. Though it was warm, it was great, sitting up there above the sparse clouds, looking down on all the world. What a thing we had done—climbing this mountain. I still have the pictures from that day. In one, she is coming up a rise and stumbling slightly, but she looks up at the camera, her cheeks flushed, a hopeful smile. She must have been twenty-two then—she looks like a little girl to me now, her whole life ahead of her. We rode the train down and then spent a few days at the beach before she left me off at my parents' house in Connecticut, then drove back to Virginia where she would go on to law school, and eventually, a house of her own, a kid, and a husband, and I would head west for adventures of my own.

Pam settles into studying her paramedic textbook. I sit there and watch the nurses crossing the street to get coffee. It's a slow day for us. Then suddenly the wind picks up and all hell breaks loose. MVAs, trees falling, calls go out all over the city. Car 453 does a call where a tree has fallen on a car, crushing the passenger compartment, but miraculously just missing the driver, who has only bruises. We are sent to an elderly housing complex where we find a fifty-seven-year-old woman who has been knocked down in the parking lot of her apartment complex by a sudden fierce gust of wind. She has fractured the orbit of her right eye and her eye is already purple and swollen shut. She is on her knees. "Lord, help me," she says over and over. "I can't see. I can't see. Why can't I see? Oh, Lord help me."

We take her to Saint Francis, which is overcrowded with patients, all rooms full, hallways, too. People with oxygen masks on, people with IV fluids running, people who look mostly dead, people who look scared, some lying on wooden backboards from motor vehicle accidents. A ragged man in four-point restraints shouts and curses: "Get me the fuck out of here, you bastards."

We do an MVA and another fall, then at six o'clock we are sent priority one for a man with chest pain in a car on Collins Street, just blocks from the hospital. A new two-door Oldsmobile has run up on the sidewalk, the front bumper touching the fire hydrant, right side against a fence. A crowd yells at us as we cross the street. "He's locked in there."

I look in at him. He is a man in his sixties in a suit and tie with an overcoat on. He is looking straight ahead. He is breathing. His eyes blink occasionally. The doors are all locked.

"Break the window, break the window," a man shouts.

When I knock on the glass, I note a small amount of eye movement to the side. "This is bullshit," I say to Pam. "It's a psych."

I hit the glass again. His eyes dart toward me, then forward again.

I keep looking at the man and start thinking. "I know this

guy," I say. "I've seen him before. I did this guy in West Hartford. We had to break into his house."

"Yeah, I was with you," Pam says.

"That's right. It's him. Look at him."

"He does look like him."

"Call HPD, tell them we need an officer so we can break the window."

She comes back and says there's one on the way.

The officer is already pulling up. "What do you got?" he asks.

"He's okay. It's a psych," I say. "He won't open up."

"I'll take care of it," he says. He takes a small metal tool, known as a window punch. He presses it against the backseat window. Nothing happens. He swears, adjusts the screw, then presses it again against the glass. It shatters. He knocks the glass away with his glove. It is a long reach to the lock, so I step in since my arms are longer. I grab a flashlight from the man's backseat and use it to hit against the lock with Pam giving me directions. "More to the side," she says, as the flashlight bangs against the automatic button. The lock pops.

I open the door and say, "Hey, how are you? What's going on?"

He keeps looking forward. I lift his left hand off his knee. I feel slight muscle resistance. I let his hand drop. It goes right back to his knee. "We're going to take you out of here and take you to the hospital," I say. I grab under his arms while Pam gets the legs. He doesn't resist and we lift him onto the stretcher. With the cop watching me, I remove his wallet from his back pocket. I look at his license. Sure enough, it is the same guy. Same name, same address in West Hartford.

"Good ID," Pam says.

"We had to break into the guy's house in West Hartford last week," I say to the cop, "and he's fine. Now we break into this car. Same guy."

The cops shakes his head. "Some world."

We get him in back of our ambulance and get his coat off and work him over. He's hypertensive, but everything else checks out. He just looks straight ahead, saying nothing. When I shine a light in his eyes, he tries to roll his eyes back into his head. "Don't play with me," I say.

I put a tourniquet on his arm and look for a vein. "Look, he's got some other IV scabs here."

"Maybe he's been into the hospital a few other times since then," Pam says.

"Where'd you get these other marks?" I ask. "You've been back to the hospital since we took you in?"

He says nothing.

"Why won't you talk to me?"

I have Pam drive on a three to Hartford, while I do the IV.

"Why won't you talk to me?" I say. "I know you're in there. What's going on?"

He sits back, his arms crossed, and stares at his chest.

I plug the IV with a saline lock, get off his legs, and check his blood sugar—normal.

He doesn't say a word all the way in. I'm thinking again: What a story. Break into his house in West Hartford and now break into his car in Hartford. Same guy. Imagine that.

At triage, I take the nurse aside and tell her the story of today and last week. She tells us to put him in room ten for a brief medical evaluation, before they move him to the psych section.

In room ten, we move him over to the bed by lifting him on the sheet, then settling him down. He doesn't look at us, holds his head down, mute.

In the car, Pam says, "The nurse thought he'd been in there a couple times this week. I think he's got some kind of major depression going on. Maybe his wife died or something."

"Maybe," I say. "I guess I was being a little unsympathetic."

"No, you treated him okay."

But I'm thinking I didn't even ask him what was going on in his life.

That night as I drive home I think about how at times I have thought of just pulling over to the side of the road and stopping, going no farther, but I've always kept on, never even slowing. I mean, what would I do at the side of the road? Who would come for me? Where would they take me? What would become of me? And how would my life ever get so bad that I would come to that place of complete despair? Could that ever happen to me?

   I still see him there, sitting in the bed in room ten, his tie on, his head tilted to the right as if he'd like to lay his head on his shoulder, but he is too tired to move it any farther, his eyes staring off.


# Presidential Debate


President Clinton is coming to Hartford. He will be debating Senator Bob Dole at the Bushnell on Sunday night. Daniel Tauber, the chief paramedic, asks me if I am available for overtime. He needs to know right away so the Secret Service can start a background check. This Sunday is my twentieth high school reunion at the prep school I went to in New Hampshire, and I have been debating whether or not I am going to go. My friend Brad, who, despite being in the middle of a hotly contested election battle for political office in Massachusetts, wants me to go, and has cleared his schedule so we can go together. Unlike him, I have never gone back. It was a hard time for me. I did poorly, and was proud just to have survived it.

   In the assembly hall they had an oil portrait of a former headmaster. There is a quotation engraved in gold at the bottom from some address he'd given to a graduating class, telling them to go out into the world and win victories for civilization, then come back to "show us your scars." Exeter was a school of achievers. The quarterly bulletin was filled with boasts of alumni about their promotions, law, medical, and Ph.D degrees received, honors and awards, children, countries traveled to, mountains climbed. Compared to them I sometimes feel an emptiness, a sense of failure like I haven't made the mark I should have.

"You ought to go," Brad says when I call him. "We'll have a good time. You're a paramedic—that's excellent. You help people. You save lives. You should walk tall in that room. And if they don't think that's great, well we don't have to hang out with anyone. We'll get a six-pack, and go sit down by the river, and tell stories."

I don't know. I just don't feel comfortable with the idea. Exeter shaped me by teaching me to lock my feelings and disappointments inside and to go on despite them—valuable lessons for a paramedic. But I don't think I'm ready to face it. Besides, now I have an excuse. Paramedic to the president. I picture myself standing just off the stage, a witness to history. Suddenly the president has a dizzy spell, he collapses. I rush onstage. The TV cameras whirl. The press snaps shots for the covers of *Newsweek*, *Time*, *People*. I apply the defibrillator, blast him. Boom. I strap the tourniquet on his arm, fire a line right. Get the flashback. Hook up the line. Running like gangbusters, as Arthur says. Fire in some epi. Some lidocaine. Sinus on the monitor. I get pulses back. The president wakes up. I help him to his feet, give him a glass of water, and he's ready to go on with the debate. Later in his State of the Union address, he recognizes me from the podium. I'm sitting up in the balcony with Hillary. I wave to the nationwide TV audience. Aw shucks, just doing my job.

I show up Sunday night at our base and find I am working with Scott Hansen. We will be a double paramedic crew. We are not covering the president. Daniel has that responsibility. Two other medics have Dole. We are to be stationed at the Bushnell, and think we will be in charge of Hillary. We drive down to the Bushnell, but all the roads are blocked off. At each checkpoint, we are sent in another direction. We end up parked by the Arch in Bushnell park, a half mile from the hall.

"But we have security clearance," I say to the officer.

"Sorry, they want you right here. You'll get called if you're needed."

We sit there for hours. I sit in the car, my legs cramped,

watching a stream of people in expensive suits and dresses with their debate tickets—purchased by huge donations—trying to get through the checkpoint, and all being sent somewhere else.

A supervisor comes by to check on us, and says not even Daniel is covering the president. They've been told if anything happens to him, they'll throw him in the limo and race up to Saint Francis, which is on alert. We're just for show.

When the debate starts, I listen for a while, but I get tired of the stock lines and phrases. I wish I smoked. I'd stand outside and have a cig and look up at the moon. I think about Brad up at the reunion. I think while the others are having drinks at the reception, he's probably walking by himself out on the athletic fields, thinking about his life, and how twenty years later he is where he is, a father of four, a husband, a man trying to make the world better, trying to live up to the great expectations placed upon him. He is a direct descendent of William Bradford, who stepped off the Mayflower onto Plymouth Rock. His grandfather was governor of Massachusetts. His father, a captain of industry. He is thirty-nine, a defeated congressional candidate, in debt, struggling to meet his mortgage, and in a tight, ugly election battle. I know he believes he can win, but the specter of another election defeat, the horrible feeling of aloneness has to be there somewhere. If he does lose, if the voters turn their backs on him, what will he do? How will he keep on fighting? Walking over those athletic fields, he will remember the boy he was, how he dirtied his jersey on the football field, dreamed the big dreams.

I think about my own life. I am not where I thought I would be—not in my life and not here tonight—a mile down the street from the big event, outside the barricade, instead of being up there behind the podium, the leader of the free world. But even though I will never be president or close to it, it does not mean that I have stopped trying to be special. So I won't be on the cover of *Time* this week. I won't get to put an IV in the president. And I suspect that if I were up at the reunion, few would look twice at me if I walked into the reception room. But I do know that if Brad and I were sitting together by the Exeter river, sharing a cold six-pack, we'd raise our beers and toast each other. Warriors. That'd be enough.

# TROUBLED MAN

*"Looking at me, I may look fine, but I got problems, I tell you, I got a storm brewing."*

# Troubled Man

We're sent to a rehab center for a man with anxiety who needs to be seen at Mount Sinai ER. A tall man in a bright blue sweat-suit is waiting at the door for us, along with an administrator in a white shirt and tie. While my partner, Mark Rozyn, goes inside to get the neccessary transportation papers, I escort the man to the ambulance and have him take a seat on the bench. I stand outside the back door. I have already teched three calls tonight, so this one is Mark's. "That place sucks, man," the man says to me. "I mean they do the detox part fine, but when a man's having the problems I'm having they can't handle it. It's about fucking time they got me out of there. I should have been out days ago. I'm a troubled man. I mean, you may look at me, and I may look fine on the outside, but inside, you don't know. You don't know. I could be like the motherfucker that done killed all those people down at the lottery. I'm sure he looked just fine till he pulled that gun out and started wasting people. You don't know what's inside. It's like nature. Nature's calm as can be, then boom, along come that El Niño. You got houses toppling, mountains falling into the sea, rainwater washing people away, hurricane, thunder, earthquakes, tornado. I feel like that inside. I got to get some help. I got me an El Niño brewing right inside, and you just don't know. Looking at me, I may look fine, but I got problems, I tell you, I got a storm brewing. I'm a troubled man."

Mark comes out of the building now with the paperwork.

"Your patient," I say.

# Sound Mind

When we arrive at the small ranch house, the policeman meets us out front and says it's a psych case. Inside, a thin, frail young woman sits on the couch. "I have diabetes," she says in a quavering voice. "You have to check my blood sugar."

"Is that all that is bothering you?" I ask.

"I have diabetes and no one will believe me," she says.

"She was just released from Hartford Hospital today," an elderly woman standing by the couch says. "She called me today to come over. She isn't well."

Her pulse, blood pressure, and blood sugar, which I take by pricking her finger and squeezing a drop onto a chemstrip, are all normal.

"You're fine," I say. "Do you live here alone?"

"Yes. I know I have diabetes. But no one will believe me."

"Well, I don't think you have diabetes. Your blood sugar is normal, but if you want, we can take you to Hartford Hospital and they'll check you out."

"I don't want to go back there. They'll put me in the psych ward. I know they will. I don't want to go there." She starts crying.

"It's okay," I say.

She is shaking.

On the table are her discharge papers from the Institute of Living. Her friend tells me that she is worried that she may try to kill herself with her pills. I try to convince the young woman that we should go to the hospital to have her checked, that we are all concerned about her.

"No," she says. "Get out of my house. I'll be all right."

"I'm worried about you," I say.

"May will stay with me, won't you, May?"

"I can't," her friend says. "You're not well. You need to go to the hospital."

"But my house is tapped. I can't stay here alone. When my phone rings there's a recording on it that says security."

"You really should come to the hospital with us." I say.

The young woman screams, "Get out of my house. Leave me alone!" Her whole body is shaking, quivering. "I just wanted my blood sugar checked. I have diabetes and no one will believe me."

We ask her what medications she is taking and whether she has taken them, and she gives us several different stories, changing each time we ask.

"Let us take you and you'll get checked out, and if everything is all right, you'll come back home."

"I don't want to leave," she says in a tiny trembling voice. "I'll be okay, really."

It goes on like this for fifteen minutes. Each of us—me, my partner, the cop—tries to persuade her to go, but we are getting nowhere. I don't think it is safe to leave her alone. I don't want to get called back for her in another two hours because she thinks she has diabetes, and I don't want someone to find her dead of an overdose the next day. She gets the ultimatum. Either she goes with us willingly, or the cop commits her and she goes unwillingly.

As much as I need improvement in many areas of the job, the one thing I am good at is getting people to come peacefully, calmly. "Come with us. We'll get you checked out, and if you're straight and honest with them, you'll get back home."

"I don't want to go," she says as we walk to the door with tiny steps. "Why can't I just stay here?"

I sit with her in the back of the ambulance. "Take me home," she says. "I'm okay, really. I am."

"You have to get checked out."

"But they'll put me in the psych ward. I know they will. Where are you taking me?"

I say, "We're taking you to the hospital to get checked. You have to be honest with them. If you talk crazy about your house being bugged or if you lie to them about your medication, then they'll probably keep you longer. You have to prove to them that you are of sound mind."

"You think I'm not of sound mind?"

"I didn't say that."

"I am of sound mind. I am of sound mind." Suddenly she yells at me. "What do you mean I'm not of sound mind? Take me home! Let me out of here!"

"Don't yell," I say. "Calm down. If you yell, they won't let you go home. Listen to me, you have to be calm, you have to be honest with them. You can't yell."

"I am of sound mind," she whispers. "I am of sound mind."

"Just be calm and everything will go fine."

At the hospital, we bring her in a wheelchair. The triage nurse is busy with two other patients. The young woman begins shaking. She starts to stand and says, "I want to go home."

But I whisper to her, "Sit down and remember what I told you. If you get up, they'll have to tie you up and you don't want that."

She sits back down. "I don't want to be tied up. I don't want to be tied up. I'm of sound mind. Sound mind."

Every two minutes she tries to stand, but I talk her back down.

"I have diabetes," she says. She tries to stand again. "I want to get out of here. They're going to put me in the psych ward. Why are they all looking at me?"

Her entire body is quivering as she stands in front of the wheelchair. I lean in and whisper in her ear again. "Sit down or they'll tie you up. Sit down and be calm. Convince them you're of sound mind."

She sits back. "I'm of sound mind. I'm of sound mind."

When the triage nurse finally comes over, I start to tell the story, but the woman stands and says, "I want to leave. I have diabetes. You'll put me in the psych ward."

"Sit down!" the nurse barks.

The woman sits and shakes in fear.

"She was released from the IOL [Institute of Living] today. We checked her blood sugar. It's fine. She's been very nervous.

She would like to go home. A friend of hers at the house expressed concern that she was going to hurt herself."

The woman tries to stand again, and again the nurse barks "Sit down!" which she immediately does. A security guard appears with restraints in hand, ready to be called.

The nurse ignores him. "Room one-oh-five," she says to us.

My partner wheels her into the room, while I go to the tech room to finish writing my report.

When I go to drop my copy off in room 105, three security guards run past me. I hear a commotion coming from the room. I think about my patient and cringe. As I enter the room, I see eight or nine guards and nurses fighting to hold a patient down.

"Goddamn, get the fuck off me. I'll kill all you bastards!" a voice growls. A security guard smacks into the wall, and a male nurse takes a blow to the nose that causes it to gush blood. I see a woman's head rise up, and snarl. "I'll kill all you bastards!" It is a large blond woman with a purple face that seems to snort smoke. The guards pile back on. It looks like a scene from a Looney Tunes cartoon, where all you see is motion and an occasional arm or restraint strap rising above the fray before plummeting back into it.

I see my patient then. She sits in a hospital gown on the next bed, her feet not even reaching the floor. She is watching the struggle with large startled eyes. She is not even looking at the meal in front of her on a Styrofoam tray: hamburger steak, potatoes and mixed vegetables, a carton of milk, and a bowl of Jell-O. "I am of sound mind," she says over and over. "I am of sound mind."

# Five White Men,
# a Blonde, and Jesus

"I want you to call the FBI," she says. She is ninety-seven years old, homebound, living by herself. "In all my years I have never seen anything like it. Five white men and a lady with long blond hair come out of that picture of Jesus. And they messing around behind the TV. You would have seen them if you'd have been listening to me, instead of trying to put that oxygen on my face and that thing on my arm. Are you listening to me? I ain't crazy. I ought to slug you."

"My partner is doing a perimeter scan," I say, "and he hasn't come up with anything yet. Still nothing, Mark?"

Mark is walking around the room with the pulse oximeter beeping. "Nothing," he says. "Clear readings. Whatever was here is gone."

"You can rest at ease," I say.

"I had a pistol I'd have shot up that wall, at least until Jesus come out. I had that picture of him since 1964. That and the picture of John Kennedy. They matching photos my daughter got for me. And Jesus, he ain't said nothing to me all that time he been up there since 1964. Then tonight he come out, he was wearing a gold crown, and he said, 'Johnnie Mae, I can heal you, but your children, and your grandchildren, and your great-grandchildren, they ain't been going to church, and we have to talk about that.'"

I stay on scene with her for more than an hour as her whole family comes over. They say she has never acted like this before. I take one of her daughters into the other room, the daughter who is her legal guardian. "I'm the seventh oldest child," she says to me, "but it's like I'm the oldest. I'm the one that always has to make the decisions." She starts to cry. I touch her shoulder.

"I know it's been hard," I say. "I don't think we need to take her to the hospital tonight. Just have someone stay with her tonight, and then maybe if she's still acting off in the morning, take it up with the visiting nurse and her doctor. She's not in danger of her life tonight. She's too old for us to take to the hospital, and she doesn't want to go. It would be too traumatic for her. I think you can wait. But we will come again if you change your mind or she gets worse."

She thanks me and signs a refusal for her mother.

Back in the main room, Johnnie Mae sits on the bed, holding her great-great-granddaughter on her lap.

"Why, don't you two look alike," I say.

"Don't you sweet-talk me," she says. "You had of been paying attention, you would have seen them, too." She says to her family. "They was here when he come in."

"I'm sorry," I say.

"The five white men was right there behind the TV along with that girl with the beautiful blond hair," she again tells the assembled family. "Then Jesus come out wearing a gold crown and speaking to me the first words he said all that time he been up on that wall since 1964. He said my children ain't been going to church, and my grandchildren, and great-grandchildren, and you know it's true. You got to get yourselves to church."

"Good night," I say.

"Good night," she says. "Have you called the FBI yet?"

"You should be safe with your family here," I say.

"Look, I told you to call the FBI. Now I ain't afraid of Jesus, but as far as those five white men and the blond girl, I want the FBI after them."

"Yes, ma'am," I say, inching out the door.

# Little Gods

His wife meets us at the door. "My husband," she says, "has a mental illness. He woke up screaming and throwing things. He's very paranoid. Could you take him to Saint Francis?"

She is in her late forties, a well-dressed, rotund woman with a soft voice. The house is an old Victorian, nicely kept. Large works of modern art adorn the foyer and front living room.

She leads us back to the kitchen where a man sits at the table smoking. He stands up abruptly. He looks like the guy in the "Far Side" cartoons who is always chained to the dungeon wall. A skinny nervous man with a gray beard halfway down his chest and long, thin hair to his shoulders. "Gentlemen," he says as his wife introduces us, "I am an artist. This is my work." He picks up a small colorful print. His hands tremble. "I call it *The Kiss of Love*. It is the third in a series."

"Nice," I say. I look at it closely. It isn't bad. It is actually pretty. Reds and oranges. It looks sort of like an upside-down heart, a red tulip, angel's wings. "You are talented," I say.

"Yes, yes, we are all little gods and goddesses," he declares, his voice trembling.

"Are these your paintings in the front hall?"

"Yes, yes, they are."

"Honey, these people are here to take you to the hospital."

"I'm not going. I refuse to go. You can't make me."

"Show me your paintings," I say. "I like that one out there."

I am looking at a colorful painting with a small quarter-sized black circle in the middle that looks almost three-dimensional in the midst of the green, yellow, and red tie-dye swirl. When I

stand fifteen feet away from it, it actually makes me dizzy.
"Here, here is the spot," I say. "Right here makes me dizzy."

He smiles. "You see well. You are perhaps, I sense, a kindred
spirit."

"It was his wedding gift to me," his wife says.

"Come, come let me show you."

"John," she says.

"Not now, honey. Let me show him."

"You did all of these?"

"Yes, I've painted all my life. When I was in school, I
couldn't write, though they held my hand and tried to make me,
but I could draw. I always could draw."

"Oh, I like that one. What a nice use of colors, the blue and
the green."

"*View from a Rock,* I call it. You like it?"

"Very much." The sea and rock are in blues, calm and
serene, the sky is green, a rolling, hurtling turbulence. A storm
brewing.

"And these," he says.

There are three pictures of large eyes with visions coming
from them. The first is a woman, lovely with three breasts. The
second a child, half human, half puppy. The third I don't understand. A horrific cloud.

"Apocalypse," he says.

"Ah, yes. Yes, I see." And I do. "Are you in museums?"

"No, but I should be. Do you think?"

"Yes, you are good, very good."

I go from one painting to the next. They are all impressive,
yet all in some way, disturbed, crying out.

"I have more in the basement."

"I'd like to see them, but we have limited time. Have you
sold any?"

"One for five hundred dollars."

"A bargain, no doubt."

"What would you pay for one?"

"I don't have much money."

"A small one?"

"The one you showed me?"

"Yes, how much would you pay for that?"

I think. "I don't know. I do like it."

"How about five dollars? Would you pay five dollars?"

"I would. Sold. You have a deal."

He smiles. "I sold one, honey. He wants to buy one."

"That's nice, dear."

I dig three ones out of my wallet and two out of my front pocket, and hand them to him. "And I want you to autograph it."

"Five dollars. Here, honey," he says. "There's five dollars." He hands it to her like a man handing over his weekly paycheck to his faithful wife.

"No, you keep it, you need to buy cigarettes."

"Yes, yes, I'll need cigarettes. Will I be able to smoke?"

"Sure," I say.

"Thank you, thank you."

I get him to sign the picture. His hands tremble, but he is able to complete his signature, and titles it *The Kiss of Love*.

He comes with us. At the door, he kisses his wife. "Take care," he says. "I love you, honey."

"I'll come see you."

"Don't worry. You take care. Lock the door."

In the ambulance, I give him my Pepsi to drink because his mouth is dry.

I asks him who his favorite artist is. He tells me he loves all artists, all of them. He talks like a boy in love, like a man blessed with a gift, with desire. His eyes glow. "All of them," he says. His eyes are wet.

# Jesus in Cedar Crest

We're transporting a manic depressive to Cedar Crest, a mental health facility, after the man has threatened the proprietor of a store on Blue Hills Avenue, calling him a money changer, and promising to return with his army of vengeance. The store owner filed a complaint with the cops, and both they and the mental health crisis team were on scene when we arrived at the patient's boardinghouse. I peacefully talked him out of his barricaded room by agreeing that he could take his Bible and religious books. The man claims he is "Jesus Christ, resurrected today in Stowe Village." He and I discuss religion. I tell him that while I do not believe in God, I am religious in my own way. While others believe in a person or force or ideal outside the body, I try to find a right way to live from inside me. When I am gone, I will be dead. But while I am alive, I want to be good, I want to stand tall, I want to be better than my human failings. "I'm not an angel, by any means," I say, "But I am well-meaning. I try hard to be good, to do what is right, to find strength inside me."

He nods, smiling beatifically at my earnestness. I'm not certain he is trying to understand me, but then again, he has that look on his face that says he understands all things. When I am finished he says, "Can you do me a favor? I can see you are a good man. I am asking you to be one of my apostles. You are going to be one of my apostles. It is ordained as so. I want you to go to television stations and tell them I, Jesus Christ, resurrected today in Stowe Village, am being held captive in Cedar Crest. I want you to tell the world what is going on. Will you do that for me?" He smiles again. "You will."

"Well, I don't think I can do that," I say uncertainly, slightly hurt that he has turned my confession to his advantage. "I can promise you I'll read the passages in the Bible you were talking about, but I'm not going to the TV stations. They'll think, pardon me, that I'm a little nutty." I hold my hands up. "No offense to you, that's just how they would view that."

"If we are going to build a kingdom on earth, we are going to have to put ourselves on the line," he says with the confidence of a minister. "What's your name?"

"Peter," I say.

"Peter? Peter?" His eyes widen, then narrow, as he assesses me more closely. "Why, you are the one who denied me. Three times you denied me."

"No, that wasn't me, that was another guy," I say. "It wasn't Peter."

He thinks for a moment. I've thrown him off guard. "Well, maybe I'm wrong."

Then Arthur chimes in from the front. "No, it was Peter. He betrayed Jesus three times."

"That's right," the man says, delighted. "You were trying to confuse me." His eyes gleam. "It *was* you who betrayed me. Don't betray me again."

"Three times," Arthur calls. "Three times."

"All right, all right," I say. "Maybe it was Peter, but I'm still not going to the TV stations."

After we have turned him over to the ward staff at the hospital and are saying good-bye, he holds his Bible to his chest and gently waves his finger at me. He recites, "'He leadeth me in the paths of righteousness for his name's sake. Yea, though I walk through the valley of the shadow of death, I will fear no evil. . . .'" Arthur puts his arm around him and joins in. They stand together, brother ministers: "'. . . for thou art with me, thy rod and thy staff they comfort me. Thou preparest a table before me in the presence of mine enemies: thou anointest my head with oil; my cup runneth over. Surely goodness and mercy shall follow me all the days of my life: and I will dwell in the house of the Lord forever.'"

"Very nice," I say, waving to them as I back away toward the door. "I'll see you guys in two weeks."

# Victor

I'm working an overtime shift and we get called to a suburban police station, where the dispatcher tells us they have a prisoner who needs to be checked out. We enter the holding area, where a police officer stands with a short male, who is pacing about nervously. "I *need* my medications, man. I *need* my medications."

"He needs to get checked out to see if he's having some kind of reaction to his medications," the officer says. "He's a little tense."

"I don't want to go to the hospital. I just want my medications. I got to take them three times a day. Man, I had them. I gave them to *you*. You lost them. They were right there."

"We're just waiting for his summons to get printed up. We're going to do a committal—or can you just take him?"

"We need a committal if he doesn't want to go."

"Yeah, okay. We're just waiting for the other officer."

I turn to the prisoner. "Can you sit down for a second? I'll take your blood pressure and . . ."

"Don't touch me. Just don't touch me."

"All right."

He scowls. "I'll roll up my own sleeve. I don't like people touching me."

"What's he in for?" Scott Dykema, my partner, asks.

"He pulled a knife on his roommate."

"I only did it 'cause he got me annoyed. You know that. He

was asking for it. He abusing drugs. I don't. I take my medications regular."

"Take off your jacket," the officer says, "so they can take your blood pressure."

"Shit!" He takes off his jacket and throws it on the table.

"Take off your shirt, too."

"My shirt. My shirt! Why?"

"'Cause I'm asking you to."

"Damn!" He takes off his shirt. On his chest is the tattoo of two manacled arms, a knife cutting the chains, and the date, June 17, 1996, on top.

"Now take off your beads."

"My beads! Not my beads! Why?"

"'Cause I'm asking you to."

"Why? I'm not going to hang myself with my beads."

"'Cause I'm asking you to."

He takes them off, shaking his head, looking like he is either about ready to cry or to explode.

He stands impatiently while my partner takes his blood pressure and I take his pulse. "What medications are you on?" I ask.

"That's a *personal* question. I'm not answering that. You're a nosy mother. I *hate* nosy motherfuckers!"

"I just need to ask you. It's part of my job," I say.

"Tegretol," he says.

"You have seizures?"

"Yes! I have seizures. You're a nosy motherfucker. I don't like you."

"Anything else?"

"Xanax. Are you done?"

"Do you have any allergies?"

"I told you I take Tegretol. Damn. You are stupid. Do I have to answer all these questions?"

"Yes, you do," the cop says.

"It's just that I need my medication. I know where it is. It's back there. It's back there. I want you to take me back so I can get it. I need it."

"You can get more at the hospital," I say. "You want to go to Hartford?"

"Hartford! Hartford! No, I hate those motherfuckers. They aren't taking me to Hartford!" he says to the cop.

"They can take you wherever you want."

"I want you to take me home to get my medication. It's right there. It's right there. I know where I left it. I need it. I need my medication."

"How's Saint Francis?" I say. "We can get you medication there. They'll check your levels and if you need it, they'll give it to you."

"Check my levels! Check my levels! All right, okay. I'll go to Saint Francis. Shit!"

"I'm going to have you step into the cell," the cop says.

He lets the officer lead him into the cell. It closes behind him but he seems to take no notice. He paces about, talking to himself. "I don't see why you even lock me up. It wasn't my fault. I just need my medication. He probably took it and sold it. He abuses drugs. He probably sold them, the motherfucker." He kicks the cell, rattling the bars.

"He gets like this when he gets tense. We've had him in a few times before," the officer says. "He just needs to get his medications straightened out."

"You talking about me—that's personal," he shouts. "Fucking cops. I hate cops."

"Calm down, Victor," the cop says. "We're just waiting on the paperwork. Then we'll get you to Hartford."

"Hartford! Hartford! I'm not going to Hartford. I hate them at Hartford."

"Saint Francis. We're going to Saint Francis," I say. "Is an officer coming with us?"

"Depends on what the sergeant says. We don't want to tie up an officer if we can help it."

Another officer comes back and says, "We're probably going to have to detain him. He's got a bad record. The liability would be pretty great. He's got a manslaughter conviction."

Manslaughter?

"Detain me. Detain me. For what? For what?"

"You held a knife to the man's throat."

"It wasn't my fault."

"I know he aggravated you, but you can't be pulling knives on people."

"Shit. I wouldn't have come with you if I'd known it was going to be this big a deal. I just need my medication. I had it, and you took it. You lost it, and now look where we are. I hate policemen. Stupid motherfuckers." He mimics, " 'Are we going to detain him or wait for the paperwork?' Motherfuckers! I hate cops!" He kicks the cell again.

The sergeant comes in. "How's he been? Calm?"

The other officer says, "A little uptight." She glances at us. "I don't think they'll be comfortable transporting him, plus the liability."

Victor paces back and forth. "I hate cops," he says. "You can all come in here and kick my ass. Just kick my ass. Bring in all your officers and beat me down, and when you're done, that's when I'm going to get up and kick your asses. Then I'm going to drag you all outside and say, 'Judge, I done this, now put me back in.' Stupid motherfuckers!" He kicks the cell again.

For the first time on this job, I admit I am a little uncomfortable with the prospect of transporting. I feel I could do it, but Victor doesn't seem stable. I might be able to sweet-talk him, but if I couldn't I don't think I could take him in a fight. I think I would just curl up in a ball, play dead, and hope he would ignore me after a few kicks and punches to the head.

They decide to transport him in the squad car. Driving back to the city, I think: I hope Arthur doesn't blow his air horn at this man if he ever crosses the road in front of our ambulance. Or if he does, I hope he's on Art's side of the ambulance.

# Restraints and the Voice

According to the father, the man has just assaulted his mother, and has been acting crazy all day. He has not been taking his medications. The man is in the other room, babbling. Does he speak English? I ask. No, Portuguese. No police officer is available. The mental health team will take at least an hour to get there.

I decide to give it a try in Spanish.

I enter the room. He turns and glares at me.

*"Hola, señor,"* I say. *"Soy un paramédico."*

He lets loose a tirade at me that I cannot understand.

I hold my hands up. *"Entiendo,"* I say. I understand. *"Pero, pienso que es un buena idea para tu va al hospital para hablar con el doctor."* But I think it is a good idea for you to go to the hospital to talk to the doctor.

He lets out another rash of angry words. He takes a hard step in my direction, like an animal getting ready to charge.

*"Entiendo, entiendo,"* I say. *"Pero pienso que es un buena idea para tu va al hospital para hablar con el doctor. Nuestro ambulancia está en la calle. Viene con nosotros, por favor."* Our ambulance is in the street. Come with us, please.

He shrugs. "Okay," he says.

I turn and he walks calmly out of the room with me. My partner, Chris Chause, looks at me openmouthed. "What did you say?" she asks.

I shrug. Some days you get lucky.

I pride myself on getting psychs to come peacefully. Countless times I arrive, and with calm voice, persuade the patient to come without a fight. It'll be okay, my friend. Come with us. My partner will drive. You and I will sit together in the back and talk. Where we are going is a good place. People will listen to you, give you a fair shake. Come.

The man speaks Spanish only. He is flushed in the face. His body is shaking. He is holding a photo in a gold frame. His mother shows me her empty pill bottles. Glyburide for her diabetes. Xanax for anxiety. She says he has taken all of them.

I stand in the doorway of the room. He looks up at me, then back down at the photo.

*"¿Qué pasa?"* I say. What's going on?

*"¡Mi bebé!"* he screams. Then looks back down at the photo.

*"¿Dónde está su bebé?"* Where is your baby?

*"No se."* I don't know.

*"Entiendo. Pienso que es un buena idea para tu va al hospital para hablar con el doctor."* I understand. I think it is a good idea for you to go to the hospital to talk with the doctor.

He glares at me. *"No. ¡Mi bebé!"*

*"Entiendo. Entiendo."*

I whisper to my partner to call HPD to find out what is taking the cops so long. While I have faith in my ability, he does seem on the verge of violence. I am not a fool.

I stay in the doorway and keep talking to him. I ask him when he last saw the *bebé*, whom I learn is with his wife. He has seen neither for two weeks. With the medication he has taken, his blood sugar may soon plummet if it is not already low. This will lead to more combativeness.

I try my patented line again. *"Pienso que es un buena idea para tu va al hospital para hablar con el doctor y las enfermeras simpáticas."* The doctor and the nice nurses.

He lets out an animal grunt, turns, and knocks over a table and a small bookshelf. *"¡Mi bebé!"* he screams.

*"Entiendo. Entiendo,"* I say, holding my hands up. *"Entiendo que su corazon es triste, pero pienso que es un buen idea para tu va al hospital ahora. Nuestra ambulancia está en la calle. Venga."* I understand that your heart is sad, but I think it is a good idea for you to go to the hospital now. Our ambulance is in the street. Come.

*"¡Mi bebé!"* He takes a step toward me.

I hold up my hands. Peace.

The cops show up, and one of them is Hispanic. He tells me to keep talking to him. Give him some time. I keep talking but make no progress. The man suddenly goes for his jacket that is on a chair. I tense, but I see he is just pulling out a pack of cigarettes. His hands shake violently. He looks around but has no match. I look to the cops. None of them smoke. An EMT from a crew that has come to back us up steps forward and lights the cigarette for him. The patient keeps shaking.

*"Venga con nosotros,"* I say. Come with us.

"Let him smoke," the cop says. "Give him time."

He smokes the cigarette.

*"Venga con nosotros,"* I say.

He suddenly smashes the picture on the ground, then walks toward us, a little too fast. He brushes against me, trying for the door. "Hold on, my friend," I say. I put my hands on him lightly. He turns toward me, looks up in my eyes. Suddenly, the little cop is on him, throwing him to the ground. The others join him. There is a brief scuffle with some close-range pummeling. The man is handcuffed, screaming like an animal.

"Enough of this shit," the cop says. "We gave him time. Let's go."

*"Por favor, por favor,"* the man cries. *"Mis manos, mis manos."* My hands, my hands.

"Tough shit, buddy," the cop says. "You had your time."

We take him to Hartford, a cop riding with us who uncuffs him when we get him on a hospital bed, where security puts soft restraints on him.

I say to my partner afterward, "I almost had him. Another five minutes and he would have been mine. I understand why they did what they did, but I would have had him."

The truth is I was surprised the cops jumped him. The cops in Hartford are truly some of the most patient people I have ever seen. They deal with unremitting abuse and are rarely provoked.

"Another five minutes," I say, "and he was mine."

\* \* \*

We're sent for a violent psych at the McKinney Homeless Shelter. Don't go in until the cops get there, they tell us.

The crisis worker meets us out front. The man we have come for is just up from Florida. He is out of control, mumbling about hitting someone, displaying violent tendencies. He was wielding a stick, and he is making no sense.

When the cops show up, one of them suggests that they ask him to step outside, so we don't have to make a scene in the shelter.

The shelter officials gradually ease him outside, giving him space. He is a man in his fifties, with a hard, wrinkled face and few teeth, his hair mussed, his clothes dirty. He looks like a man who has been doing some hard traveling. He sees the cops and the health workers, who form a semicircle around him, with no one closer than twenty feet. His eyes look right and left, then they meet mine. I step forward. *"Señor,"* I say, *"Me llamo Pedro. Soy un paramédico. Entiendo que su está cansado por su viaje. Vengo conmigo. Vamos al hospital. Hay comida caliente allí."* I understand that you are tired from your trip. Come with me. We go to the hospital. There is hot food there.

He says he has already eaten. He does not want to go.

I step closer. I hold my hand out. My voice is right on pitch. There is no one else in the world, except the two of us. We are just two poor workers of the earth. Life is hard and our hearts are often sad. Come with me, and we will share our burdens together, *compadre*. The only thing to fear is the fear of being alone, unloved in this vast cold world.

He comes to me like a child to candy, like a tired sinner to a priest, like a drone to a hypnotist. I hear one of the cops remark, "That was easy." I hear someone else say, "That was great."

En route to the hospital, we talk. He babbles a rush of words. He meant to hurt no one. They were trying to hurt him. A man in Florida took his money and tried to lay the blame on him. He is innocent, he declares. When I mention medicine, he gets agitated. No, he will not take it, it makes him feel ill. I continue to speak calmly. He is in my care, under my spell. I am the voice.

At Hartford Hospital, I guide him through triage and back to the psych room. I give my report, then say good-bye. You are a good man, I tell him, they will take good care of you here. I walk out and stop at the triage desk to talk with Alison, one of my favorite nurses. Over the intercom I hear, security to 105. The guards go rushing past. "Oh, no," I say.

"Your friend?"

"I hope not."

I feel like a betrayer sometimes. I get them to come, get them to trust me, and then at the hospital, they strap them down. There is a fight, a struggle. Do they blame me? Do they remember me as good? A friend? Or I am evil? The seducer?

Back in the car, I tell my partner, "I hardly ever need restraints. If you're calm, and you use your voice, you can get them to go peacefully."

The very next call. Not the next day or two calls later: the very next call. Vanity takes the fall.

Unresponsive, Franklin Avenue. Third floor. Hurry, the cop says. A nineteen-year-old girl sits in a chair, her head down, drool coming from her open mouth. She is pale with black hair over her eyes and a tattoo of a dead flower on her neck. She passes the hand-drop test. Her pupils are pinpoint. She barely breathes. Her mother says she has taken a bottle of the mother's Xanax, a depressant. Does she do heroin? I ask. Yes, the mother says. She doesn't look a hundred pounds. I think about just picking her up in my arms and carrying her downstairs, working her in the ambulance, getting on to the hospital. I think there is more going on here than just heroin, more than just a blast of Narcan will fix.

My partner gives her a deep sternal rub, shakes her shoulders. Her eyes open, and she stands up, startled, off balance. I grab her by the shoulders to keep her from falling. "Get away from me," she says. "Leave me the fuck alone."

"You need to go to the hospital," I say.

"I think not," she says. "I think not." Her words are slurry and she totters.

"No, you really need to go."

"Fuck off," she says. She swings at me. I grab her wrists and hold them. She kicks at my shins. I manage to avoid her thrusts. I start in with the voice, quickly. "It's okay," I say. But I fear I have already lost her. She looks at me with disgust.

I want to soothe her, I want to say, sweet, sweet girl. You may think the world hates you, but I see the beauty in you, the sweetness at your center. I want my words to wrap around her like a lover's arms, hold her, warm her, drift her off, make her feel secure. Let the voice hold you.

"You fuckin' bastard," she screams. "Unhand me, I know my rights. I know this tune. Been there. Done that." Her black fingernails are out like cat claws, but she can't break loose from my grip.

"Calm down, my friend, it's okay. You don't need to fight. We want you to be okay. We want you to be all right."

"Then leave me the fuck alone."

"How many pills did you take? I need to know."

"I didn't take any. I'm sober as my tits."

"Okay. Did you do heroin tonight?"

"Fuck you. I know my rights."

"You're going to the hospital," the cop says. She breaks one arm free from me and turns to claw him. He grabs her from behind. I grab her legs and we carry her kicking, screaming, and clawing down the stairs.

"Let me go," she screams. "I'm calling the cops. I know my rights."

"He is the cops," I say, as we go out the front door. "And he is going to handcuff you if you don't stop kicking."

"Oh, I'm sure. I'm sure."

We get her in the back of the ambulance, seated on the bench seat. She has stopped fighting for the moment but still refuses to cooperate. I tell her I need to get her to lie down on the stretcher so I can take her blood pressure and give her some medication. This immediately sets her off again, and now the four of us, my partner and I and two cops, are wrestling with her, tying her arms and feet to the stretcher with pillowcases. She is spitting and clawing and kicking. "Your mother sucks cock for crack!" she screams.

"Holy shit! Where's this blood coming from?" the cop says, and immediately lets go of her arm. She clocks me in the face. I grab her hand and press it to the stretcher. The pillowcase around her wrist is absolutely soaked through with blood.

"She's got HIV," the cop says. "Be careful. I know her. She prostitutes herself."

I try to figure out where the blood is coming from. I think she must have cut herself on the stretcher, but I can't find a mark. I remove the soaking pillowcase and see a deep horizontal gash at her wrist that is bleeding profusely. Holding her arm down with my knee, trying to avoid her biting me, I wrap a trauma dressing around it. It turns out it is a week-old scar from when she tried to slash her wrists.

We finally get her tied, and she lies there, glaring at me as if I am evil itself. I meet her stare as I tell my partner we can go to the hospital now. I am soaked with sweat, my glasses have been knocked off my face, I can only imagine what my hair looks like. Still staring at her, I take my jacket off, then open the biotech. I take out a three-cc syringe and a bottle of Narcan.

"What's that?" she asks.

"Narcan," I say.

"What are you going to do with that?"

"I am going to stick you with it."

"No, you're not, like hell you are."

I don't think I really need to give it to her. I know she has done some heroin, and there is always the possibility of her nodding back off. She probably has also done some cocaine, that excited her once she was aroused. The 1.2 milligrams I draw up will wipe out what is in there. It might even make her puke. I draw it up deliberately. I feel like a principal taking out the paddle, the executioner tying the rope or loading the gun.

"Don't," she says. "Don't you stick that in me."

I think: You bitch. My words meant nothing to you. You knocked my glasses off, spit in my face, insulted the memory of my mother, and worse, exposed my vanity.

I jab her in the shoulder with the syringe. She screams and breaks loose from one of the restraints. I plunge the syringe in, but she knocks it loose and we wrestle over it. She is about to bite my neck when I slam her with my shoulder, knocking her chin away. I grab the syringe and toss it out of reach. I get hold of her arm and retie her.

She spits and again insults my mother.

"You can be more original than that," I say.

She pants and then I feel the fight go out of her. "I feel sick," she says.

"It'll pass," I say.

By the time we reach the hospital she asks to look at the wound on her arm. I untie her arm and show her. She nods sadly.

"I did that a week ago," she says.

"Can I take your blood pressure?" I ask.

"Sure," she says.

I mark down the pressure and her pulse. I tell her we're going in, and she needs to stay calm. She nods. I leave the one arm unrestrained.

At triage Alison looks me up and down. "What happened to you? You look like a wreck," she says.

I tell her the story. Alison looks over at her and says she knows her. She's been there before. She assigns her to room eleven.

In the room I tell the girl, as staff comes in to help, that we can go through the whole routine again—the fighting, kicking, clawing, spitting, swearing, wrestling—and the result is going to be the same. She is going to end up on the other bed, so please (sweet girl) just move over for us peacefully when we release the restraints.

"I know my rights," she says. "I'm checking myself out."

One of the male nurses says, "Let me handle it." He tries his version of the voice. A poor imitation of mine, I think. "So what do you say, just move over for us," he says.

"I think not," she says.

"Put your gloves on," I say. "Watch out for the spitting. Don't take personally what she's about to say about your mother."

I step away. Their show.

As soon as I am out of the room, the battle begins. "Your mother sucks cock for crack!" More security race into the room.

I go and sit in the back EMT room to write up my report.

"What were you saying about restraints?" my partner says.

"Don't go there," I say.

I call dispatch for times, and Susy gives them to me, then says she wants me to take one out of room 105 going to the Cedar Crest psychiatric hospital, a man in restraints. The same guy we brought in earlier. "Great," I say. "I sweet-talked him into coming peacefully, and they tied him up. He's going to be happy to see me."

"Is that a problem for you?" she asks.

"No, I'll face it," I say. I know they're short of cars and I'm right there.

The nurse in 105 says we may need restraints. He was a wild man, she says. If the medication wears off, you best be prepared. I look at him. He is all doped up on Ativan, sleeping. En route to Cedar Crest, I keep the lights dark in the back. He doesn't even know I'm there. He mumbles, tosses a little, trying to get comfortable. I watch over him. Rest, I whisper. Sleep. He turns on his side, tries to find comfort. The words come softly. The voice. Golden slumbers fill your eyes. Zippity, hombre, do not cry, and I sing a lullaby.

# RECOGNIZE

*Who is shaping them, nurturing them, directing them, loving them? And even those who get love and direction, what will happen to them in the world they live in?*

# Girls

The call is for difficulty breathing on Nahum Street. We pull up, get out carrying our equipment, and head toward the building. Several high school–age girls are watching us. One shouts, "How come you ain't running? She having a hard time breathing. You run. You hear me, you run."

We keep walking toward the building.

"You run or I'm going to kick your ass. You hear me?" They laugh.

We knock on the door. It opens and in the room there are another eight high school girls, all laughing.

"Who's sick?" I ask.

"She is, she's got asthma."

A girl, maybe sixteen, sits in a chair, a little short of breath. I listen to her lungs and hear a slight wheeze. "What happened?" I ask.

"I was fighting and I got short of breath. It happens every time."

"You fight a lot?"

"No, but I always get short of breath when I do."

"You should look at her, she got cut," another girl says and points to a shorter girl with a shirt that's cut open near the breast.

I look at her while Art gets a treatment going for the girl with the wheezes.

There's a superficial cut on the top of her breast. "She was trying to take my babies off," the girl says. The others all giggle. "Look at Keshia's nose, she the one hurt the worst."

A girl comes out of the kitchen holding a wet paper towel on

111

her nose. I have her remove it and there are deep jagged teeth marks there. "What happened to you?"

"Girl bit me. That Kamona, she always biting. Second time that bitch bit me. Last month she took a gob out of my arm. She nasty that way."

"She always biting," another girl says, "that's her style."

"She got you good this time." Another girl laughs. "She latch on to your nose and hold on like a pit bull."

They all laugh and giggle.

"How many of them were there?"

"Just three," the girl with asthma says, "but when we jumped them, they all got knives, so they whipped us this time, though Karisse come away with one of the knives."

The police come to take statements, and the girls identify the other girls, but readily admit they were the aggressors because one of the other girls was flirting with Latisha's boyfriend.

"He don't even like you, Latisha, look what trouble you causing everyone," the girl with asthma says, and they all laugh. The girl starts coughing, she's laughing so hard. Arthur and I and the cop just shake our heads. None of them end up going to the hospital.

"The youth of today," Arthur says as we walk back to the 471.

# Fidel

A man doing yard work across the street shouts at the woman who has come to the door to let us in. "What are you doing? What kind of trouble are you causing now?"

"The boy is sick," she mumbles as she lets us in. "The boy is sick."

Inside the house it is sweltering. There are three children sitting in the front room. We walk into the kitchen. Steam rises from four huge pots on the stove. All the windows are closed. It has to be over a hundred degrees. The sick boy, a nine-year-old, is kneeling in the bathroom, trying to vomit.

He is pale. He looks up at me, expressionless.

I hear shouting. The man from across the street is in the kitchen. "Woman, I'll send you to the hospital," he says.

"Come with me," I say to the boy. I want to get him out of the house.

In the kitchen, the man is still shouting at the woman, and she is muttering, "The boy is sick."

"Where are you going with him?" the man says to me. "Everything is all right here. He just has an upset stomach. No need for the ambulance."

"I'm just going to take him outside where it isn't so hot, so I can check him out. No big deal," I say.

He looks at me suspiciously.

"I'm just going to check him out," I say. "Are you his father?"

"No," he fumbles. "No."

"She his mother?"

"No, she's just watching him."

"Okay, I'm just going to check him out."

It is a relief to be outside. I call on the radio and ask for a police officer.

The boy nods when I ask him if he is okay.

"What's your name?"

"Fidel," he says, looking at the ground.

"Who are these people?" I ask.

He shakes his head again like he doesn't know.

"Where are your parents?"

He shakes his head.

I slowly get the story from him, though he volunteers nothing. His mom dropped him off at a baby-sitter's and the baby-sitter dropped him off here. He doesn't know where any of them are and he has not eaten since last night. He doesn't know any of the other three kids either. He sits on the grass looking down at the dirt. The cop comes and I tell him the story. He goes in the house.

"You want something to drink?" I ask the boy.

He looks at me and says nothing. He reminds me of a wild animal, starving, but uncertain whether to trust a man.

I take a fruit juice out of my small cooler and open it up. I hand it to him, but he won't take it. I put it on the ground. "Go ahead, drink it."

He picks it up, takes a sip, then puts it back.

"Drink," I say.

He has a few more sips, then sets it down.

The cop comes out of the house. There are beads of perspiration on his head. "It's hot in there," he says.

His sergeant shows up and starts questioning the cop about what he has done. Then they both go in and talk to the woman.

I stay out there with Fidel. "Drink," I say. He has a few more sips, then sets it back on the ground but still eyes it.

The cops come out with the other three kids marching behind them like ducklings. The woman stands at the door watching. "Come on, boy," the cop says to Fidel. "We're all going down to the station."

He follows slowly.

"See you," I say.

He doesn't turn.

# No Kin of Mine

We're sent to a call in a public housing complex. In the yard, Arthur points out the carcass of a small dog against the building. Flies circle about it. It has been there long enough to smell.

"These people," Arthur says. "Can you believe that?" Kids are playing nearby. "What a shame," he says.

In early 1995 the governor of Connecticut, John Rowland, appoints a new commissioner to the Department of Children and Families, and pledges to wipe out child abuse in the state. The deaths and abuse cases keep coming: child rapes, deliberately inflicted burnings, abandonment. In 1997, the emotionally drained commissioner resigns for personal reasons. The governor acknowledges the problem may take longer to solve than he believed. He appoints the agency's chief critic, the head of the office of child advocacy, as the new commissioner. The new commissioner declares, "I want the families to be treated like my family. I want the children to be treated like they were my own children."

Nice sentiments, but how do you translate that into action, into something real?

We get called for a maternity with complications in Stowe Village. On the third floor, a woman seven months pregnant complains of abdominal pain and cramping. She looks like hell. "I was up all night," she says, taking a drag on her cigarette.

"Can you please put that out?" Arthur says.

She crushes it out on the top of a beer can.

"Do any drugs or drinking?" I ask.

"I had a couple beers and did some base."

"Oh, that's good for your baby."

She glares at me.

At the hospital, I give the report to the nurse in labor and delivery. "She was up all night, drinking and doing crack," I say.

"I didn't do crack, I did base," the woman says.

"Big fucking difference," I say.

The America I grew up into believed in the Horatio Alger myth. Any kid could become president. America was red, white, and blue, number one. If man could walk on the moon, he could do anything. Right wrongs. Cure sickness. Stop war. Government service meant serving your country. Being good and decent. Doing for the U.S.A., not for you. And all that noble rhetoric.

Nowadays I try not to even watch the news. If it isn't boiler-plate campaign ads proclaiming Mr. Dudley Good Citizen as a miracle worker and Mr. Snidely Opponent as a plague-ridden-pusher-down-the-stairs-of-old-ladies-in-wheelchairs, it's boilerplate spin written in interchangeable cut-and-paste out-rage or acclamation. I just get tired of all the posturing. Day after day of the Clinton-Lewinsky scandal drags on. Did he have sex with her in the specific definition? Did he commit per-jury? Did he try to get her a job? Did he try to obstruct justice? Was he entrapped? I listen to both sides till I want to scream. Day after day. No end in sight.

Two things I know. The life kids in the inner city are born into is a disgrace to everything this country stands for, and it seems the politicians aren't even on the same planet.

We are in the elevator of the Sands apartments, a crummy ten-story apartment building off North Main Street, next to the Bellevue Square housing project. The elevator stinks of urine and jerks as it goes from floor to floor. We were sent for a drunk and found a jaundiced man lying on his side on the mattress in his bare apartment, his pants stained with dried urine. A friend of his was concerned about him and called us, but the patient didn't want to go and we couldn't make him. He wasn't drunk; he was lying in his own apartment; he knew what day it was. He just wanted to be left alone.

The elevator stops on the third floor and two little kids get on. They look like brothers, the older probably seven. He holds the younger, maybe four, roughly by the neck.

"What's your name?" I ask.

"I don't talk to strangers," the older boy snarls. He whacks the head of his brother, who is smiling at us, and forces him to face the door.

"We're not strangers," I say. "My name is Mufasa, and this is my trusted friend, Riffiki."

He looks at me with disgust. In his eyes I see nothing but

hardened—*I've had enough bullshit in my life*—disappointment. "You ain't no Lion King," he says.

The door opens on the first floor. He pushes his brother out, keeping hold of his shirt.

I watch them trudge down the hall.

I remember back when President Reagan was shot. There was an NCAA championship basketball game on that night, and there was some controversy over whether or not they should play in light of the day's tragic events. They asked one of the players what he thought about the issue of playing that night, considering the president was lying in the hospital with a bullet wound. The young man—a black kid from the ghetto—allegedly answered, "He ain't no kin of mine." There was a lot of outrage made over his statement, which was an offhand comment in the locker room. At the time I thought it was bad; a college basketball player ought to be more sensitive and respecting of the position of the president. But thinking about it today, what these politicians are doing in Washington is similar. Don't you think you ought to quit playing political games and do some serious work out of respect of the position of children in America? And it's like the whole Congress is saying, They ain't no kin of ours.

# The Corner

I'm reading this book called *The Corner* by David Simon and Edward Burns, a journalist and a retired detective who spent a year hanging out in a drug-ridden inner-city neighborhood in West Baltimore. I bought the book to see if it would give me an insight into some of the people we deal with. The book depresses me. I see enough lives destroyed by drugs that much of the book is information overload for me, but what I find fascinating is the authors' description of how the drug trade changed over the years from a highly organized and disciplined venture into the street-corner chaos that exists today. They claim it was the introduction of crack cocaine in the early 1980s that changed everything.

Crack cocaine is cheap, plentiful, and you can't ever get enough of its rush. You don't need a syringe to get high. It begins with a pipe or a snort up the nose. It may lead to the syringe and a speedball mixture of heroin and crack, but its initial appeal brought in the young mothers who'd been squeamish about heroin and needles. Families started falling apart. Kids running wild. When federal law enforcement efforts had put the older dealers in prison, the new line of dealers started using kids to carry their stash. The dope was so potent, the dealers started using themselves. Soon everyone was cheating everyone. Crew members stealing from each other. Mothers stealing their kids' stashes. No one could trust anyone. Before crack, violence was punishment for specific infractions of rules. After crack it was a by-product of emotion or gesture. With prison overcrowding, fear of arrest was little deterrent. With a hundred dealers on the street, the herd provided protection. The cop cars roll up, everyone runs. Even the weak who are picked off are back out on the street in no time.

The authors write:

The old code of the dealers is useless now; the new rules are different and have to be.Because, by necessity, any new logic must allow for a mother to stand on Monroe Street and tout Red Tops with her two-year-old in tow. It must allow for a fiend's theft of the television set from the recreation center, of chalices from the corner churches, of the rent money from his mother's bedroom. And the rules of the corner cannot stand if they prohibit a thirteen-year-old from holding up a single vial of coke and telling a playmate with brutal honesty that for one of these, your mother will step up and suck my dick.

* * *

The book is a vivid account of how our inner cities have become a wasteland of the disenfranchised. It doesn't offer much in the way of solution, but I really wonder if there is one, at least one simple and catchy enough to garner popular support. You have some serious history and time to undo here.

It's three in the morning. An icy, rainy night. I drive down Edgewood Street. A man in a hooded black sweatshirt wanders out of an abandoned house. Two men stand against a fence, fading into the darkness. Up on the corner, a boy stands, hands in pockets, eyes alert to the oncoming traffic. Any hour of the day. Any weather. Always there.

# Mother

She is in the bathtub, fully clothed, soaking wet. Her son, a boy of fourteen, is patting her face, calling her name, pleading with her to wake up. Two smaller children watch from the bathroom door. An old woman gets them away.

I can see the track marks on her arms. The surroundings of the house look familiar. I think I have been in this spare apartment before, for this same woman.

"How much did she do?" I ask the boy. He says nothing. I look at her pinpoint pupils. Heroin. "I'm not the cops," I say. "How much?"

"A couple bags, I think," he says. "She doesn't tell me."

She is breathing four times a minute. "Don't throw water on someone like this." I say. "It'll just give her a cold."

"She wouldn't wake up," he says.

"It's okay. We'll take care of her."

I put the tourniquet on her arm, look hard for a vein. Her arm

is familiar. I know I have treated her before. I remember the
tattoo of the butterflies and the names Maria and Anna in-
scribed under each. I got the IV the last time right above the
butterflies' antennae. A hard stick. Nothing doing this time. I
can't find or feel a thing. Screw it. I draw up the Narcan. I will
give it to her IM, intramuscularly. It will take a little longer but
will get the job done. I roll up her sleeve and see another tattoo,
a heart with the name Roberto under it. I swab it with the alcohol prep, then, feeling poetic, jab the needle right into the
heart, push the Narcan in.

"Mami, Mami," the boy says.

"Give it a couple minutes," I say. "She'll come around."

He looks at me, uncertain.

Arthur takes the gear down and gets the stair chair.

The woman's breathing is picking up. She opens her eyes
and is groggy. She coughs, then throws up on herself.

"Mami, Mami," the boy says.

"We're going to take you to Hartford Hospital," I say.

She looks at me, then up at her son, then at the neighbors in
the doorway to the bathroom. She closes her eyes.

"Mami, Mami, are you okay?" the boys asks.

She rubs her head with his hand but says nothing.

We carry her out in the stair chair, down the hall, past the
neighbors' open doors, down the old wooden stairs. I look at
their eyes, the neighbors, old women and kids, young men.
This is a familiar sight. An overdose. An ambulance.

The boy comes with us.

At triage, the nurse recognizes the woman and says, "You
were here yesterday." She shakes her head and asks me for the
name for her chart.

I look back at the woman and her boy. He rubs his hand
against her face. Fourteen years old. His mother lies there,
eyes closed. She's thirty and looks fifty. "What's your name?"
Arthur asks the boy.

"Roberto."

# Childhood

They say the seeds of the man are in the child. I am looking through some old papers when I come across my kindergarten report card.

INTELLECTUAL DEVELOPMENT
*Sense of Humor*
Generally good—likes humorous incidents, very adverse to teasing
*Interest in Stories*
Very interested
*Interest in Conversation*
Normal interest, can carry on a very intelligent conversation
*Reasoning*
Exceptional except during occasional streaks of anger
*Purposeful or Random Activity*
Purposeful

EMOTIONAL DEVELOPMENT
*Temperament*
Generally even with occasional streaks of emotion, conscientious, strong-willed
*Ability to Face New Situations*
Has shown no fears or worries
*Independence in Work and Play*
Sufficiently independent in both
*Kindness, Responsibility Toward Others*

Very kind and responsible as a rule with occasional
impulsive response when angry
*Self-confidence*
Appears sufficient

## PHYSICAL DEVELOPMENT
*Large Muscle Coordination*
Sufficiently developed
*Small Muscle Coordination*
Crayon and pencil sufficiently controlled
*Ability to Relax*
Sufficient
*Dressing Habits*
Dresses and undresses self
*Speech*
Distinct

## SOCIAL DEVELOPMENT
*Cooperation*
Cooperative as a rule but will occasionally choose not to
do as others; separates himself occasionally from others
*Leadership*
Has shown leadership qualities in his ability to plan
activities, courses of action, a good organizer
*Ability to Follow*
Has the ability to follow, but will quite often attempt
to change plans with a little original idea of his own
*Reliability*
Dependable in the right place at the right time, comes
when called
*Defense of Own Rights*
Very good at reasoning his differences with others as
a rule but can become very emotional on occasion
*Consideration of Others*
Takes turns, is polite

I think that report card is remarkably accurate to this day.
While I can cite major factors in my later life that shaped me

in one way or another—in high school, not able to be a leader, I chose not to be a follower; not getting into Harvard as my relatives had made me question my self-worth, but enabled me to choose a nontraditional path; discovering literature, and then striving to live up to it, to be a worthy companion of its heroes; having few close friends, but holding them tightly; disappointing myself occasionally when love was on the line and I chose self-survival, but feeling all its cost—they didn't change the essential person I am.

I am basically moral. I am generally even-tempered, but I do get pissed off every now and then. Still, I am polite, and as the report says, I come when called. I had parents who cared about me, who gently kept me in line and tried to show me the straight path.

I wonder about these kids in the city, from birth to five: who is shaping them, nurturing them, directing them, loving them? And even those who get love and direction, what will happen to them in the world they live in? Some days I think if I had been a black kid living in Hartford then I would have easily gotten into Harvard, but then I think that's ridiculous. What I achieved was achieved with advantages. What would I have become if I had grown up with a drug-addicted single parent in the inner city? Would I be a kind drug-dealer, a considerate gang member, an impulsive thief? Would I be writing this book or instead would I be sitting on the cold floor of some crack house, entertaining my doper friends with dazzling tales of capers and thievery, as I used my IV skills to find the last hidden vein in their withered arms and scarred necks? Would I even be alive?

# French Fries

The mother meets us at the door. She is maybe nineteen years old, a huge beefy girl, wearing an apron with a name tag that says CHANEL. She is crying. The call was for a small cut to a child, but her tears have me wondering. She leads us up the stairs, then disappears behind a huge straw curtain that separates two rooms. She comes back holding a tiny little girl in her huge arms. The girl has a small cut to the side of her face. It has stopped bleeding but may need a stitch or two to close. "I just come to pick her up after work and she playing, and she got pushed into the bed frame. I knew something was wrong. Her friend Taimika said, 'Tay, I'm sorry, I didn't meant to hurt you, Tay.' They both named Taimika. I saw the bleeding and I got so worried, and I give her this towel." She starts crying again.

"Calm down," I say. "She'll be okay. Hey little girl, what a pretty little girl, you are." She has the most beautiful smile, and her hair is neatly done in cornrow braids. I hold her in my arms. She can't weigh twenty pounds. "She'll be all right," I say.

We take them to Saint Francis. I have the little girl on the stretcher. Her mother sits on the bench leaning over her, still wiping her eyes. The girl looks up at her, eyes wide open, uncertain, bordering on fear. The mother cries, her voice breaking. "I'm sorry, Tay, Mommy loves you. Mommy loves you." Her beefy hand caresses her daughter's cheek. "Tay, Mommy got you dinner but she left it at home. Mommy got you french fries cause Mommy knows you love french fries. Mommy loves you, Tay, Mommy got you french fries."

I have this vision of the little girl eating nothing but french

124

fries for the next ten years until she is as big as her mother, and has a child of her own, whom she, with all the love in her great heart, can give french fries to.

"Mommy loves you, Tay, Mommy loves you."

# Social Club

It is 2:54 early Sunday morning when we get the dispatch. "Four-seven-one, respond priority one for the shooting."

We are just blocks away from the address—a popular north-end social club. We race down Woodland while three cop cars, their lights whirling up Homestead, swing in, fishtailing behind us. It feels like a scene right out of a movie.

Car 601 is also dispatched. "They're saying there are three people shot," Suzy Ribero, our dispatcher, says.

The club is ahead on the right. Cars are parked up and down the street. A mob of people running out of the building. Chris Carcia, my partner, parks in front. I get out, grabbing the green bag. The scene is chaos. "Who's shot?" I ask.

"In dere, in dere, mon!" a man shouts. The crowd is dressed all in white and black, dresses and evening suits. I look to the front door and see a man running out toward me, gesturing angrily. "Run, mon, run! He's hurt bad!"

Chris and our rider are pulling the stretcher out. The crowd is glaring at me. Someone grabs my arm and yanks. I swing my arm loose. "Easy," I say. I start toward the door. I walk deliberately. I need to be careful, alert.

"Get the fuck in here, mon. He's shot bad," a young man with a glistening bald head and an earring shouts at me.

I keep coming. As I go up the steps, the crowd that has been running out seems to stop. They swing around me, sweeping me up, rushing me in. I see a blood trail on the foyer floor, leading out. "Who's this from?" I ask.

"He already left. The man's hurt bad, inside."

Women are crying. The men look angry. The second entrance door slams shut; I can't open it. The crowd around me starts to beat on it. The crowd inside turns and rushes back and opens the door. "You stand there and hold it for my partners," I shout at a woman as I am pulled forward.

"This way, mon, this way!"

I am taken down a hallway, following the blood trail. I can see another crowd gathered around what I presume is the victim.

"Clear way!" I shout. "Clear way!"

"He got a pulse. He still got a pulse. He going to be okay. He going to be okay," a man shouts.

The victim lies against the wall. He is a young man in his twenties with a goatee, nattily dressed. He is not breathing. He looks like a man laid out in a coffin taking a nap. I touch his neck. Nothing. I pull back his vest, find a bloodstain on his right lateral chest. I turn and look back for my partners. All I see is the black-and-white dressed wall of people pressing against me.

"Who else is shot? Is anyone else shot?"

"No, just him, just him."

"Do something, mon! Do something!"

"Back off. Make way. My partners are coming. Give them room."

I turn back to the victim. I notice a champagne bottle by his side. I pull out the ambu-bag from the green bag. Chris comes through with the stretcher.

"We have a traumatic arrest," I say. "Let's get him up and out of here."

We lower the stretcher down, start to lift him. Several people try to help us. We flop him down, pop the stretcher back up and head for the door. I throw in a few compressions. Our rider bags. We wade back through the crowd, shouting at them to part. At the doorway the stretcher jams. We spin, pivot it, while a cop manages to unhook the second glass door to give us maneuvering room. The light of a videocamera held above the crowd shines on us. We race to the ambulance, lift him in back.

"We need a board under him," I shout to Chris. "Let's get his clothes off and get him on the monitor. I'll get the tube."

I pull out my airway kit, go in with the laryngoscope. I can barely see the cords. I ask for cric pressure, but my view is obscured. I see a hole but no cords. I pull out, and bag for a moment. I look to my left and see heads pressed against the window and the glare of cameras. I go in again but see nothing. The back door opens and it's John Burelle from 601.

"What can I do for you, Pete?" he asks.

Chris does CPR. The patient is in an idioventricular rhythm on the monitor. Only the lower part of his heart is working, but is slowing rapidly to an agonal, dying rhythm. My rider is going for an IV line.

"Drive to the hospital," I say. It's just blocks away. "Drive and patch."

I throw the laryngoscope aside and plunge my hand into the man's mouth. With my fingers I feel the soft epiglottis, the piece of flesh that guards the vocal cords. I lift up on it, then pass the tube between my fingers, using the tips to turn the tube upward, and feed it into the trachea. I feel the slight vibration in my right hand as the balloon at the end of the tube rubs against the bumpy cords. I'm in. I yank the stylet out. I inflate the cuff, then quickly tie on the mouth holder. "Where's the ambu-bag? I need the ambu-bag."

"It's at your feet," Chris says.

I grab it, attach the end to the top of the tube. I ventilate. It compresses easily. I have Chris squeeze, while I listen. Positive lung sounds. Nothing over the belly. I'm in.

"Go, man, go," I say to John, who is in the driver's seat now. We're out at the hospital a minute later.

They have a full trauma room staff waiting for us. I give the report. "Shot through the chest. In one side, out the other. Not breathing when we found him."

"How long has he been down?" the doctor asks.

"Ten minutes, five minutes, not long, but probably long enough."

I step back as they take over bagging and compressions. They throw some epi down the tube and put in two chest tubes. I have the rider stay to watch while Chris and I walk down the hall. She goes out to clean the ambulance and I get a run form and sit down. The waiting room is mobbed as everyone from the club has come down the street to find out what is going on. I'm on the phone with Suzy, getting my tag and times when I start hearing a woman cry, "Oh Lordy Jesus, oh Jesus, oh God, oh Lordy Jesus!"

"What's all the shouting?" she asks.

"They must have just told his mother," I say. "The waiting room is packed with people from the club. It's a mob scene."

I drop my paperwork in the trauma room, where the young man lies naked and motionless on the gurney, two chest tubes sticking out of his side, blood on the floor, the ET tube sprouting out of his mouth. Only two staff members are still in the room, finishing the recording notes. On the table, I see his effects—car keys, a beeper, wallet, some change.

I collect my crew, we get in the ambulance, and get the hell away.


# Recognize


The eighteen-year-old muscled male was brought in for altered mental status, smoking crack and drinking. He is put in the crisis unit, where they take his clothes and dress him in a hospital johnny. He is reluctantly cooperative, if sullen. Then his beeper, which is in the bag with his clothes, goes off. The ER tech won't let him have it. The young man becomes combative and a security alert is called. He kneels on the bed, breathing

hard, his muscles flexed. The guards stand around him, latex
gloves on, straps in their hands, ready for the word to move in.

"Don't you disrespect me," he says to the tech.

"You can't have your beeper," the tech says. "Now sit down
and calm down."

Another tech touches his shoulder. He knocks the hand
away. "Don't touch me. Now gimme my clothes."

The guards step closer, but his chest expands and the veins
in his neck bulge. They step back.

"Listen! You got to recognize my rights!" He is breathing
hard. "Recognize! Recognize! Recognize!"

"You're not getting your beeper. You're in the hospital now."

The other tech moves closer and he whirls on him. "Don't
touch me." The guards pounce on him. The tech puts an elbow
into his throat and a knee hard on his chest. He is strapped
to the bed. Overwhelmed, contained, he lies there, breathing
heavily, muscles tensed.

"Act like an animal, you get treated like an animal," one of
the guards says.

The young man's eyes burn with rage.

# Sterling

Two kids are playing basketball in the street in front of a
makeshift hoop attached to a telephone pole when we pull up
in the ambulance. Each looks to be about ten years old.

"Who you looking for?" a fat shirtless kid says. "You looking for Sterling? Everybody looking for Sterling. Sterling live
over there. Up the stairs. You come for Sterling, right?"

We walk up the creaky stairs of the dilapidated house and go
in through the open door. There is Twenty-Love graffiti on the

ceiling. Twenty-Love is the gang that makes the north end
its home.

On the second floor landing is a broken window; there are
drips of fresh blood on the floor. A handwritten sign on the
door reads: "Do not knock. Do not even think of coming in. Do
not in any event try to disturb."

We go up to the third floor and knock.

"Who dere?" a voice demands.

"Ambulance," my partner says.

The door opens. A short, barrel-chested young man stands
there. "Second floor. You looking for Sterling. I call the ambulance for him. He got beat up and he need to get checked out.
He waiting for you on the second floor."

My partner and I look down the stairs at the sign on the door.
"You want to call him for us?" I say.

"He waiting for you."

We walk hesitantly down the stairs, and standing to the sides
of the door, knock on it. There is no answer.

My partner knocks again this time with the radio. "Ambulance!" he says.

Still no answer.

The guy comes down the stairs, and also standing to the
side, shouts, "Yo! Sterling, man! Ster-ling!"

The door opens a crack and a tired-looking woman in her
forties stares at us.

"Ambulance," I say.

"They looking for Sterling," the guy says.

"You've got to go up the other stairs," she says. "His room
on the other side."

"We're here now, why don't you let us through," my partner
says, stepping in. We walk through several rooms, each sepa-
rated by a curtain, each a different home. In the back room next
to the bathroom, a tall, muscular, bare-chested man looks out
the window. A woman rubs his shoulders.

"Yo, Sterling, man. It's the ambulance," the guy says.

Sterling turns and looks at us. He has a gash on his forehead,
his face is bruised. He is holding his hand in a bloody towel. He
says nothing, just nods and walks toward us. The woman stays

behind. We walk back through the other rooms, their tenants eyeing us silently. "Excuse us," I say.

As we come out, the two kids stop their basketball game and the fat one says, "I tole you that's where you find him. That's where you find Sterling."

Sterling steps into the back of the ambulance with my partner, as I go to the front to drive.

At the hospital, the nurse sits him in the triage room, then cleans the dirt from the scrapes on his hand, chest, and head.

My partner tells me the story Sterling told him. A young man from the south side heard a north-end guy named Sterling was pushing his mother into a life of drugs. He and two of his buddies piled into a car and came looking for "Sterling." He was the first Sterling they found. It didn't matter that he was the wrong one.


# Heroin


Going up the stairs, I think I have been here before. I know I have. There is a constant feeling of déjà vu on this job. The addresses and the calls meld together, but you sense the familiar: a dog outside on a chain, eye-catching graffiti on the wall, a couch in the hallway, the same neighbor.

She is lying on the single bed, eyes open, dilated. Oh, man. Cool to touch. Rigor in the jaw. The needle on the bed, inches from her hand. "No," I say to my partner, who has the radio to his mouth to call for backup. I look at the tattoos as I put her on the monitor. The butterflies, the heart. Flatline.

"Where are the kids?" I ask the neighbor, the old woman.

"Took away," she says.

I stand there in the spare dirty apartment. A world in disarray. I can smell the garbage. A cop arrives, and we turn the scene over to him. We walk out carrying our gear. At each doorway in the hall, people watch us leave, taking no one with us.


# Darkness


At home I sit up in the dark. I think about the city—the streets I work—this world.

I think sometimes what I'd like to do is get a great giant syringe and fill it with Narcan. Then drive it deep into the ground, into the city's heart, down where the waters lie. Push it all in. Clean out the whole system. Chase the bad medicine away. Then in the morning the water will run fresh out of the faucets and give the city's tired soul, all of us, a new start.

# BODY COUNT

*Where the tension lies is not in the day-to-day call, but in the long-run view. What is this doing to me?*

# Dead Man's Poker

We get sent for an unknown. When we arrive, a man who does not speak English points up a set of outdoor back steps that lead up three flights. I grab the $O_2$ bag and monitor and follow him up the stairs. We go into a small kitchen, where several people are sitting around a table. There are beer cans on the counter and on the table, where they have been playing cards. "Who is sick?" I ask. *"¿Dónde está el enfermo?"*

The man points to a man sitting against the wall. I look at him for a moment. He is sitting up straight, his elbows on the armrest of the wooden chair, his hands on the table, still holding his cards. His eyes are closed, and his complexion is gray. While I am looking at him for only a split second, it seems like I am staring at him for ten or twenty seconds. This man is dead. He is not breathing. He is completely motionless, like a wax figure. I grab him and whirl him down onto the floor, and shout at my partner, Marisa Monnaccio, to call for backup. The woman at the table immediately starts screaming, which sets off the others. The man is flatline on the monitor. Marisa starts CPR while I intubate him and fire a milligram of epinephrine and one of atropine down the tube to try to jump-start his heart. The room fills with people, all screaming, crying. The fire department shows up to help us carry him downstairs. The woman throws her right arm across her forehead and does a swan dive to the floor.

"You need another ambulance for this lady," a firefighter says.

I glance at her, and her eyes open briefly, then close. I say, "She'll be all right."

"Is he going to be okay?" one man asks, as we lift our

patient up on the board, still doing CPR, never anything but flat line on the monitor.

"No, he's dead," I say.

The woman, who has revived herself, screams, and faints again.

We work him all the way to the hospital, and they work him about ten minutes there, then call it.

I have no idea how long he was sitting there at the table—probably about five minutes, given our response time. They must have gotten concerned when he was taking so long to play his cards. A final long look at the hand he'd been dealt.


# Storm Inside the Calm


Paramedics and EMTs can, in the midst of an emergency, appear to be the calmest people on the planet. Race lights and sirens to a call ten times a day and, after a while, you learn to nap on the way, so long as you're not the one driving. Or like in the famous car chase scene in *The Blues Brothers*, while Jake and Elwood are racing through the shopping mall being pursued by the cops, they comment on the mall's stores and wares. Enough shootings, cardiac arrests, diabetic comas, and it becomes pretty routine. Where the tension lies is not in the day-to-day call, but in the long-run view. What is this doing to me? Does what I am doing matter? Does anyone care? Do I? And what will become of me when I can no longer do this? A bland job? An obnoxious boss? The path to death. Arthritis in my bones. Bloated legs. Sick at the heart. Fluid in my lungs. Blue lips. Faceless EMTs coming through the door. An IV in the arm. Mask over the face. A tube down the throat. Vomit. V-fib. Shocked. Flatline. Pounding on the chest. A rough ride.

Sirens fading out. Left on the table. Lines pulled out, but ET tube still in place. Rolled down to the morgue.

# Asthma Code

We're covering downtown when we hear the call go out—asthma on Kensington Street in the north end. They give it to 875—a basic car. "They'll call us if they need us," I say when Arthur looks at me as if to suggest we offer to take it.

Ten minutes later we hear 875 on the air asking for a medic. The dispatcher says, "I don't have any nearby. Are you loaded? Just go to the hospital."

"We need a medic," she insists. "She's really bad."

Arthur, radio in hand, is about to volunteer us, when the dispatcher calls. "Four-seven-one, Kensington Street for the asthma."

"We probably should have just taken it the first time," I say.

"No, they should have dispatched us."

We're several minutes away. Maybe a minute less with Arthur driving. Asthma can be frightening as people gasp for breath, the airway passages in their lungs narrowed and plugged with mucus from the sudden onset of the disease. Our standard treatment is to give them a Ventolin breathing treatment, .5 cc of Ventolin mixed with 1.5 cc of saline water dropped into a plastic nebulizer chamber and hooked up to an oxygen line that turns the mix into vapor the patient inhales. We tell the patients to take deep breaths through the mouthpiece. If they are too weak to hold the nebulizer, we can fit the container into a $O_2$ mask that we strap to their heads. They receive nonstop treatments until they clear up. If they are really bad, we can call for orders to give subcutaneous epinephrine. I always start an IV line: fluid moistens their dried-out lungs and loosens the mucus. At the hospital, they can use the IV access to give steroids to further open up the patients' breathing.

Asthma is a common call in the city, particularly on dry, cold days like today. A lot of people let their medications—little pocket Ventolin inhalers—run out, or they overuse their inhalers so they're not effective when a real attack comes on. Sometimes the panic is almost as bad as the disease, the fear that they can't get a breath. The first thing I do is listen to their lung sounds. In an active asthmatic I usually hear a high-pitched teakettle sound as the air tries to force its way through the narrowed bronchioles. I listen not just for the sound, but for the quantity of air being moved. A high-pitched wheeze is better than no sound at all. No sound means no air getting through.

We pull up on scene and 875 has their back door open, their patient already loaded. I grab the blue bag, which has the $O_2$, my airway kit, and the nebulizer setup in it. I get in back. One EMT has the ambu-bag out and is trying to ventilate the patient.

"She's stopped breathing," she says.

The patient is a woman in her thirties. She is pale, cyanotic, and still as death. I reach for the red airway kit and open it up. The EMT tells me the patient was gasping for breath when they got there and they had to drag her outside. The family said she had been getting steadily worse all day.

"Get the monitor," I shout to Arthur. I unzip my airway kit, pull out a number seven tube, slide in the stylet, attach a ten cc syringe to the end. I grab the laryngoscope that has a number-four curved blade in place. "Get out of my way," I say to the other EMT. I kneel down by the head of the stretcher. I put the blade between her teeth, sweep the tongue to the left, and lift up. I have to get the tube. The light illuminates her throat. I can't see anything. I lift higher. Still nothing. I pull back. Nothing. She needs air right away. I don't want to pull out. I have to find the cords. Come to me, come to me. Wait, I see white, but no opening. It's the cords. They are closed shut. I have never seen this before. I lose sight of them and pull out. I grab the ambu-bag and try to ventilate, but I'm not getting much air movement. With the cords shut, her trachea is closed off. She's not getting any air into her lungs. I have to get air in.

I go in again. I lift up. I still can't see the cords. "Give me some pressure," I say to Arthur.

He pushes down on the cricoid cartilage just below the Adam's apple, where the cords lie. They should drop into view, but I'm not seeing them. I pull back some on the blade. I see them again, still closed. I pass the tube into the mouth, and angle it down toward the cords. I twirl the tube, but keep hitting low. I can't get them to hit against the cords. I swear. I pull the tube out, reconform the shape with the stylet, then go back in. I see the cords. I bang against the white and feel something give way. "I think I'm in," I say hopefully.

"I didn't feel it pass," Arthur says.

That is bad, but I try to ignore it. Maybe he's wrong. I inflate the cuff, a small balloon, which secures and seals the tube in the trachea. I get the ambu-bag ready. I secure the other end of the tube with the tube holder, a bite block that tapes around the head with Velcro. Arthur connects the ambu-bag. He squeezes it while I listen over the lungs with my stethoscope. I hear lung sounds on the right. "Positive." I hear them on the left. "Yes!" I listen over the stomach. I hear sounds. I swear I'm in, but I don't know. I didn't feel it pass. I look at the balloon on the end of the cuff. It is not inflated. I may have torn it, while passing the tube. That could explain the air escaping into the stomach. The trachea is not sealed off. But maybe I'm in the esophagus. If I'm not in the trachea, she's in serious trouble. She may already be done for. I swear and yank the tube out.

"Ventilate," I say. I disconnect the ambu-bag from the tube, but the mask has fallen to the floor and I can't find it. I need to reattach it to the bag. I've got it. I fumble to get it on.

"We need to start CPR," Art says. He has her on the monitor, and she is in an agonal rhythm, just a few complexes. He starts thumping on her chest. I am trying to get up but am wedged between the stretcher and the wall. I am losing control of the scene and the patient. It's all going horribly wrong. Arthur shouts at one of the EMTs to take over compressions. He forcibly lifts me up, frees me. The family is in the front of the ambulance. If we had left right away, we'd be at the hospital by now. I made the decision to work her on the spot because she needed it right then, but I haven't delivered. I bag, but not much is getting through. I grab the laryngoscope, a fresh tube, and go in again. I can't see anything. Then I think I see the cords, so I go in with the tube.

"I didn't feel it," Art says, but I shove it through. I listen. I hear lung sounds right. Lung sounds left. I listen over the belly. Air sounds. Fuck. I yank the tube. I feel hopeless. Give me the minutes back. Let me start again. I want to quit. I wish I'd never been on this call. I grab another tube, set the stylet. "Last time," I say. She may already be gone, but the same decision holds. I decided to make my stand here and I have to live with it. She needs the tube now, not in seven minutes at the hospital. Now.

I use the three curved blade. There are the cords. There is a slight opening. I pass the tube, pushing through. "You got it," Art says. "I felt it that time."

Lung sounds right. Lung sounds left. Over the belly. Nothing. "Yes." I'm in. I look at the monitor. All she has is the wavy rhythm of CPR.

"Stop CPR," I say.

The line goes flat.

"Start CPR."

I grab a sixteen-gauge needle from my pocket and jab it into the jugular vein in her neck. Blood flashes back into the chamber. A direct hit. I hook up the line. It runs flush. I need a dressing. The EMT hands me one and I tape it down. We switch positions. Arthur takes over bagging. The EMT goes to do CPR. "Watch out for the line!" I see it before it happens. Her boot gets caught in the line and the line pulls out of the IV. Blood flows from the woman's neck onto the floor. I grab the line spurting fluid, and reattach it to the catheter which fortunately is still in her neck. I open up the Biotech and grab the pouch of epinephrine, and popping the yellow caps off, one after the other, start firing the ten cc vials through the line. Epi after epi. With a couple atropines thrown in. "Let's get out of here."

We're finally on our way. The tube's good. CPR is in

progress. I've got the line, and I'm slamming the drugs. "Come on back," I say. "Come on back!"

I glance up at the monitor, and I see something funky. It's like CPR, but with little notches. I slam more epi. The rhythm changes. "Stop CPR."

I've got a rhythm back. "Feel for pulses."

Arthur feels her neck. "Nothing," he says.

"Keep going," I say. "CPR."

I put more epi in. Her color is starting to pink up. The monitor is changing again.

The driver hands me back the mike and says the hospital's on.

I give a quick report. "Approximately thirty-year-old female asthma code. Was in respiratory arrest, now in cardiac arrest. We've got her intubated, a line in, and starting to get some movement on the monitor. Be there in five minutes." I toss the mike back to the front, not even waiting for a reply.

"Stop CPR. Check pulses."

Art feels her neck again. "I've got something. I've got a pulse."

"We saved her?" the EMT says.

"We've got a pulse," Art says.

Her heart is beating wildly at 160 on the monitor in a rapid A-fib. She's back, but I'm not celebrating. I fear we are too late.

We wheel her into the hospital, and right into the cardiac room. I give my report. "Any trouble with the intubation?" the doctor asks.

"It was very hard," I said. "I got it on my third attempt."

"Did she get ventilated? How was the resistance? Was she breathing when you got there?"

"She was out when I got there. The cords were closed."

"Laryngospasm," he says.

Arthur congratulates me on our save as I walk out of the room, but I shake my head.

She goes to intensive care. A few days later I go up to see if I can find a nurse to talk to. She tells me our patient, Nicki

Joyner, is hemodynamically stable, but had an anoxic event—anoxic meaning a period where insufficient oxygen caused tissue death. Her heart is beating and she is breathing on her own, but she is unconscious.

I tell myself I didn't give her asthma. I didn't delay calling 911 when she started having trouble breathing. I came as quick as I could. I didn't cause her cords to close or cause her to stop breathing. She wasn't breathing when I got there. But I think, Christ, if I had only gotten the tube on that first attempt. If I could only have gone in, lifted up, seen the cords, passed the tube, heard the lung sounds on the left, heard them on the right, no sounds over the stomach. Got her ventilated. Forced the $O_2$ in. Maybe. Maybe she'd be back at work today or home laughing with her family around the dinner table. I lost her. Then I rallied, seized control, and brought her back, but to what end? I know other medics have told me about codes they've done, where they've brought the person back, gotten the save, and now instead of the person being six feet under the ground, they're in some nursing home, hooked up to machines.

I talk to people about the call. The veteran medics and doctors cringe when they hear asthma code. These are people who shouldn't die. Asthma is a preventable disease. But people abuse their medications, they don't call when the attack starts, so when the medic gets to them, or when they are brought into the ER by their screaming family, they are on the edge—savable, but the window is short. I feel like a wide receiver who gets his number called late in the big game. I get open, the pass hits me square in the chest, but I drop it. It can mean nothing or it can cost the game. I catch the next pass, dive and grab another, but it's too late. I'm a yard shy of the goal line. I didn't get the tube right away and that was it. Season over.

Two weeks later, we're sitting outside Saint Francis when the call comes in for a person unresponsive on a back porch on Barber Street, not far from Kensington.

"It's a drunk," Art says. "Whaddya bet?"

"Or a code."

"Yeah, that's right, the last one we had unresponsive in the hallway was the big guy, facedown with his shorts around his knees. Stiff. Remember that guy?"

"It's a code," I said, "I've got a feeling. It's a code."

"Four-seven-one," the HPD dispatcher calls.

"Four-seven-one."

"Four-seven-one upgrade to priority one. It's a pediatric respiratory arrest."

"Four-seven-one, copy," I say, then, to Arthur, "Fuck."

All the way there I am concentrating on what I am going to do. I'm going to get the tube. I'm going to get air into that child. I am going to bring that child back to life. I will not, I cannot, I must not fail.

We pull up and there is a woman standing on the corner flagging us down, crying. "Around back, around back," she shouts.

Arthur pulls the stretcher and I grab the blue bag and monitor. We run down the drive to the back door. A man stands behind the glass. I try to open the door, but something is blocking it. "You can't open it," he says, crying. "She's blocking it."

I look down through the glass and see a body facedown.

I turn and run along the side of the house. Wendy Albino and Matt Lincoln in car 463 pull up on scene to back us up. I scale a low fence and go in through the front door. The house is dark. "What happened?" I ask a woman, who is wailing and following after me as I run.

"It's my baby. She got asthma. She's not breathing."

"When did she stop?"

"I just found her. She been gone two hours."

I get to the back and find her in the stairwell of the back breezeway. It is cold there. She lies facedown wearing a heavy snow jacket.

"She's not breathing," the man says, through his tears. "We thought she'd gone to school."

I touch her face. It is cold. I try to move her jaw. It is stiff. She isn't breathing. Fuck, she's already dead. Rigor has set in, I think. But she's a kid. I'm going to work her anyway. I reach down and put my arms around her, and lift her up forcibly. I fall against the door, and, as it suddenly gives, we tumble out onto the back driveway where the stretcher is set up. My equipment isn't there, nor is Arthur. He and the other crew come charging out of the house behind me. I lift her up onto the stretcher. "Let's just get her in the truck. We'll work her there. Get the ambu-bag out," I shout.

"Is she breathing?" Wendy asks.

Matt undoes her jacket. We wheel her toward the ambulance.

"Wait, she's squeezing my hand," Wendy says.

Matt feels her throat. "She's got a carotid pulse."

None of this is sinking in. It makes no sense to me. We lift her in the back. I go for my airway kit. I see the woman from two weeks ago lying there on the stretcher. Not breathing. I remember the struggle to get the tube, to get air in her. I've got to get the tube. I've got to get the tube.

"She's breathing," Wendy says.

I grab her jaw, and her eyes open suddenly.

"I don't think you're going to need to tube her," Matt says.

The girl smiles at me and says, "Can you get my mommy?"

I let my laryngoscope drop to the floor.

We all sit there.

"I'll get her mom," Wendy says.

Arthur puts his hand on my shoulder.

I am all at once too tired to even move. On another day I might want to pick this girl up and spank her. I might want to put a large needle in her arm to teach her a lesson for her cruel, attention grabbing charade, but now I am beat through and through. Spent. I let out my breath. I sit there.

It is a week before I feel like doing anything for anybody.

# Gory Stories

One of the most common questions any EMT gets from a layperson is "What is the goriest thing you've ever seen on the job?" Very few of our calls are what you'd call gory, but that's what everybody seems to think about what we do—gore, be-headings, guts hanging out.

A mechanic at the garage where I'm getting my car inspected sees my uniform jacket in the backseat and says, "I bet you must see some pretty gross stuff, huh?"

"Yeah, I guess, a little bit," I say.

"Like what, tell me. What's the most gruesome thing you've ever seen?"

I think for a moment, uncertain whether I want to get sucked in or not, but he looks so expecting, I tell him, "I guess it'd have to be this body I saw spread-eagled on the road at an MVA scene. Completely ripped open. I could see the intestines, the heart. It stunk something fierce."

"Yeah, aw, gross," he says.

I don't tell him the body was that of a skunk, run over by a station wagon that swerved to avoid the animal and ended up crashed into a telephone pole, leaving the driver with a facial laceration and some back pain.

"What else?" he says.

I think for a moment, then come up with a real call. I tell him about the guy shotgunned to the groin. "He was lying there holding the bloody mess, and there was nothing but a bloody crater."

"Did they fix it?" he asked.

"That's what he was asking, all the way to the hospital, 'Is it going to work? Is it going to work?' I gave him an IV and told him it was going to hurt a little, and he said, 'Anything so long as it'll work.' "

"Well, did they fix it?"

"Yes, they did. He can even pee through it, though it's a couple inches shorter than it was before."

I can see the pain on his face. He squeezes his legs together. "What else, tell me one more. You get any other good dead bodies?"

I tell him about the guy in Bellevue Square where we're called for a possible 78—a dead body. We arrive outside the complex, and I have to say the air smells a little odd. The cops have been waiting for us to arrive. They say no one has seen the gentleman who lives in the first-floor apartment for two weeks, and there is a funky smell coming from his apartment. The apartment is dirty. I can hear a TV coming from the kitchen. I walk in slowly. Roaches run before my feet. I pass the kitchen. The small black-and-white TV is playing, the local weatherman is giving the forecast—hot. I pass the bathroom. Empty. The back bedroom lies ahead, the door is open. I hum to keep from inhaling the odor that is wafting out to meet me, hovering at my nostrils, begging me to breathe in. I walk slowly, like a soldier through a mine field, ready at any moment to take cover or run. I step through the door, look to the left, and there he is, a four-hundred-pound naked man, bloated up like a pig, lying on his back, a chair broken to the side. There is shit or dried blood, some dark brown-black material all over the floor. My eyes are fixed on his scrotum—it is the size of a football. The smell is in my nose now, and I fight back the heaves. He has a thick black beard. Bugs run out of his mouth.

"Bugs?" the guy goes. "He had bugs running out of his mouth?"

"Bugs," I say.

I turn and walk past Art. I go into the kitchen, and fight back the heaves. The cop looks at me from the door. "He's dead," I say.

I am supposed to put a monitor on all my dead bodies and run a flatline strip for documentation, but I just head out the door. The only place he's going to come alive is in my dreams. I go to Saint Francis and scrub my mustache. For days every now and then I get a whiff, and I cringe.

The mechanic is impressed. "You must get a lot of chicks, huh, being a paramedic?"

"I get my share," I say.

"Cool," he says.

"Yeah," I say.

I start to collect gory stories from other medics to impress the guy with when I go back—tales of transected bodies, beheadings, kittens eating dead bodies' eyes, the intestines hanging out of a guy I treat who was stabbed while buying drugs, intestines that looked like deflated sausages. But before I get back the mechanic goes over to his friend's house one night, has a couple beers, and they start passing a gun around. It goes off unintentionally and shoots him through the neck. A bloody scene. He's DOA at the hospital.

# Too Much Confusion

*Carbon monoxide is a colorless, odorless gas present in the fumes of gasoline engines. The deadly gas binds with the oxygen-carrying molecules on red blood cells and prevents them from transporting oxygen to the tissues. Symptoms can include nausea, headache, faintness, and confusion. Continued inhalation can lead to death.*

The call comes in for a car running in a garage. The address is a town-house complex. A woman stands outside a one-car garage, under an apartment, frantically hailing us. As we get out I can hear a car engine running inside. A man runs toward us and goes to the door, hands shaking, to key it open. As he lifts the door up, I can see a tube running from the tailpipe into the back window of the car. The small garage is filled with smoke and fumes. I can see a body slumped behind the wheel. A man runs past me and opens the car door. He tries to pull the person out, but the person is stuck.

"Give me a hand. I can't get him out of here. He's stuck!" the man shouts at me.

I hear fire engines approaching. I know the garage is filled with carbon monoxide, but they are only fifteen feet from me; the man is shouting, pleading for my help. "Get the stretcher," I shout to Arthur, then I run in. I grab the man, who is unconscious, under the arms and pull. He comes loose. The other man grabs his legs and we have him out. We carry him toward the ambulance as Arthur lowers the stretcher.

The man is shirtless and looks to be in his twenties, a muscular Puerto Rican kid. His skin has a yellow hue, his face is cherry red. He is not breathing. We set him on the stretcher and lift it quickly into the back.

"Get him on the monitor," I say to Arthur, as I reach for the airway kit.

I grab the laryngoscope and a number-eight tube. I go in, lifting up on the tongue. The cords drop down into sight. They are huge—they look like the entrance to a cave. The light at the end of the laryngoscope blade illuminates the cords as if they are onstage, like they are talking to me. Here I am, baby. Tube me, tube me.

I pass the tube easily. I tape it down, check for lung sounds. In solid.

"He's flatline," Art says, starting CPR.

I have the drug box out. I take out a bristojet and a vial of epinephrine. Holding one in each hand, I pop off the yellow caps with my thumbs. The caps float up in the air, spinning.

"Where's the fire department?" Arthur asks.

"Why don't you stick your head out and get somebody?"

I screw the epi into the bristojet, separate the ambu-bag from the tube, squirt the drug down the tube, reattach the bag, give two hard squeezes on the bag, then reach over and do some compressions, as Arthur gets out and shouts for someone to help us. A cop gets in the driver's seat as Arthur gets back in with me.

"Where are we going?" the cop says.

"Hartford Hospital," I say.

"How do these lights work?"

I lean toward the front and flick them all on. "Go nuts," I say. He grins like a little boy, shifts into drive, and we're off.

I need to get an IV line now. The kid has a huge external jugular (EJ) vein running down the left side of his neck. It is so big, I think I could lay it across a mountain stream and walk across it like Karl Wallenda. I take out a fourteen-gauge needle and stab it with an audible "Ya-haa!" I get a flashback. In. I hold pressure on the neck, withdraw the needle, and attach a line of saline Arthur has spiked to the catheter.

"Gangbusters," Arthur says as we open the line up.

We are flying through the streets now. On one bump, both of us end up sprawled across the patient. Arthur shouts at the driver. "A little easy on the gas," I say.

The cop smiles, like the dog Mutley who used to drive Dick Dastardly's racing machines.

I fire epis one after the other into the line. Arthur's doing CPR. I bag. We whirl around another corner and go flying again. I find my eye looking at that other external jugular vein on the right side of his neck. It's calling to me. Stick me. Stick me. I take out another fourteen and go for it. "Ya-haaa." I get the flash.

"Bilateral EJs," Art says. Impressed.

We have two bags of fluid running wide open. I am still firing epis in. Still flatline on the monitor. We hit a bump and go airborne. We crash over the patient. I feel like I'm in a rodeo. "Bag for me while I call the hospital," I say to Arthur.

I lean into the front. As I reach for the C-Med mike, I say to the cop, "Good driving."

I call C-Med and am connected to the hospital. "Approximately twenty-year-old male in cardiac arrest, found in a car in a garage, engine running. Tubed, two lines running, asystole on monitor. See you in a couple minutes."

I go back to firing epis through the line. As we pull into the hospital, I fire my last one.

We wheel him right into the cardiac room. I see one of the nurses looking at me a little strangely as I give my report. "Four atropines, twelve epis, no change. Got an eight tube." I point to the EJs. "Two fourteens." They check the tube placement—solid—hook him up to their monitor, asystole. The nurse is still looking at me as I strut in place.

"Six-eighteen," the doctor says, calling him.

I get our times from the office. We arrived on scene at 6:00. He was declared dead at the hospital eighteen minutes later. Unbelievable time coming from where we were.

I am all fired up. I don't know if it's getting the tube, bagging the double EJs or the wild ride, or just that it's the end of the week for me. I feel sorry for the guy, but the call went great, couldn't have gone much better. While Arthur is resupplying, I put the stretcher back together. I lift it up to put it in the back of the ambulance, but I can't get it to lock. I keep slamming it against the lock, but it won't catch.

Eric Salisbury, a longtime EMT, is standing there watching me with a bemused look on his face. "Typical paramedic," he says. "Doesn't even know how to put the stretcher in. You're putting it in backward, buddy."

I look at the stretcher. Son of a gun. "Hey, I'm tired," I say. "End of the week."

I take it out, turn it around, and finally get it to lock.

When we clear the hospital, Arthur says, "Nineteen years old. A permanent solution to a temporary problem." He shakes his head. "What a shame."

The Red Sox game is on the radio. First inning. Mike Stanley drives one deep. It's off the center field fence. A double. Two runs scored.

"Yes! Yes!" I shout, pounding the roof of the ambulance. "Sox! Sox!"

"You all right?" he asks.

"Yeah, no, actually, I have an incredible headache."

"Yeah?"

"It's killing me. Long fucking week, huh?"

"We were busy."

I feel really spacey. The spaciness you get when you are real tired and can't concentrate.

At the base, we shake hands. "Good job on the code," Art says.

"You, too. We did great. Have a good weekend."

"Drive safely," he says.


To get home I take I-84 east, then get on the flyover to I-91. I've got the game on, but I'm not paying attention to it. I'm just driving through the night, watching the red taillights, the highway signs. I live in Enfield. I normally take exit 48. I know something is wrong when I look to the right and see the lights of Springfield ahead. I've gone five miles past my exit, clear into Massachusetts. I used to live in Springfield so I guess I just tuned out for a bit. I get off the exit and get back on south-bound, getting off at exit 49, Route 5. I head south. I see the light up ahead is red. I go right through it. I wasn't supposed to do that. I go through the next light. Cars are honking at me. Another red light is ahead. I'm not certain what to do. I think about pulling to the side of the road, but instead I go through the light. Three red lights, man, that's not right. Fortunately, my right turn is up ahead. I take it, and go straight down Alden street, which runs right into my parking lot. I get myself parked and get out. Safe.

The hallway down to my apartment seems awfully long. I get into my apartment and get a beer and turn on the stereo. I hit random play on the one hundred CD changer and up comes Jimi Hendrix, "All Along the Watchtower." I sit on the couch, and pick up an old newspaper, but my eyes can't focus. Too much confusion. The words scroll across the page. *Guitar.* I sense something wrong. I fear I am poisoned, mother. The giant cords. The Karl Wallenda veins. The pounding in my brain. The red lights that couldn't contain me. I am weary. No relief. I see a series of fast black-and-white flashing photos of my life. Faces of friends. Faces of patients. A skeleton in a black hood laughing. I want to lie down, but I float upward.

The disorder, beer bottles, dirt, and grime ground into the carpet. Flashing lights. My world. I bounce against the ceiling like a balloon.

# I Don't Want to Die

The eighty-year-old man is passed out on the hardwood floor just outside the bathroom from which he exited. He is cool and clammy. We are unable to get a pulse or blood pressure. I put him on a nonrebreather. On the monitor he is going at 24. En route to the hospital I start an IV and give him a milligram of atropine and run the bag of saline wide open. His rate comes up to 52, but still no pressure. I am thinking I may have to tube him, though his family told me he wants no extreme measures.

"I don't want to die," he mumbles now, surprising me. "I don't want to die. I'm not ready." He is crying.

After eight hundred ccs, I get a pressure of 90. I ease the fluid off. His pulse is still in the fifties, but I can palpate it. The crisis has passed.

At the hospital, when his family visits, he is alert and they say he is more coherent than he has been all day. They thank me. "You saved him," his daughter says to me.

"Just doing my job," I say.

Driving home, I hear his voice over and over, the tears in his eyes, the words, "I don't want to die, I don't want to die." The words crowd around me like the night that has fallen. I feel cramped, closed in. I want to drive back into time, whipping around the globe in my car at a hundred times the speed of light, chasing old sunny blue-sky days at the beach, coconut buttered bathing teens and cut muscles I never had, going back to when I was young and didn't know about any of this—this getting old and dying, this end.

# An Ordinary Head

I'm working the Sunday overnight with Toniah Abner. It's been snowing all night, and we've done nothing but B.S. accidents, cars skidding into one another, people with neck and back pain, insurance talking. It's cold and windy out, and I only have one glove, can't find the other. We finally get a break around four A.M. We sit in the front of the ambulance, the heat on, and doze. I think I hear our number called. "Four-seven-one?"

I answer. "Four-seven-one."

"Four-seven-one. Motor vehicle accident on Maple Avenue. On a two."

I nudge Toniah.

"Another MVA," I say.

"Great," she says. It is a half hour before our crew change.

Maple is only a few minutes away. The streets are still snow-covered, and we can't go more than thirty. Ahead we see two cars in the middle of the road. The back of a white car and on the other side, a Jeep. The doors to the white car are open. Two people stand in the road waiting for us.

"This is going to be B.S.," I say.

As we pull up, Toniah looks back at the white car and sees the windshield is smashed. "Well, maybe not," she says.

The cars hit head on. The hood of the white car has been bent upward. The Jeep doesn't have too much damage.

"Are you okay?" I ask the man who comes limping toward me.

"Yeah, I'm all right. You should check him out though. I don't think he's doing so good."

"He's got a nasty cut on his head," the woman says.

I walk over to the car. There is a grapefruit-sized hole in the windshield. The man is sitting in the front seat, his head slumped forward.

"Hey, buddy, are you all right?" I ask.

He doesn't answer.

I give his shoulder a little shake. His head falls backward, his mouth open. A grim bony smile. I shiver. He has a huge gash across his forehead. He looks like he has been scalped. I look at his chest. I don't see any movement. He doesn't look like he is breathing. He is not breathing. I shout, "Toniah!"

We extricate him quickly from the car.

"Is he breathing? Is he all right?" the woman on scene asks.

I say nothing as we wheel him past her to the ambulance and lift him in the back. Toniah gets out the ambu-bag and monitor as I quickly open my airway kit. I go into his throat, lifting the tongue, looking for the cords. A gush of blood comes at me, but Toniah reaches up, and presses down on his throat, dropping the cords down into view, and blocking off the blood. I pass the tube and quickly secure it. He is flatline on the monitor. Toniah starts compressions. A cop opens the back door. "Get in front and drive!" Toniah says to him.

Two minutes later, we are out at the hospital and charging into the trauma room. The man has a torn aorta. When they insert a chest tube, blood gushes out. They work him five minutes, then call it.

We go back to the scene to look for my trauma shears, which I find on the icy ground by the car door. We look at the cars. There is more damage than I thought. The Jeep is extensively damaged under the bumper. The white car seems to have veered across the road. The engine is pushed in a foot or more. The steering column is bent. I look at the hole in the windshield. There resting on the glass, half in, half out of the car are a pair of gold wire-rim glasses.

\* \* \*

I'm working with Manny Sandoval. We get a call for a motor-cycle accident just blocks from the hospital. Thirty seconds later, HPD calls for a second ambulance, saying it's really bad. It doesn't take us a minute to get there. I see a bike wiped out on the sidewalk. A woman moaning nearby. I start toward her when a firefighter—the accident is right across the street from the fire station—says, "Go to him, he's really bad." She looks at least alert. I turn and approach him. He is sitting up, his back to me. He turns and looks up at me. His face is a bloody Hal-loween jack-o'-lantern. His eye is on his cheek, hanging out of its socket, bouncing with the thrashing of his head. "How are you?" I say stupidly, then shout, "Manny, C-spine."

"Gloria, Gloria," the man calls.

The fireman is telling me he hit the curb and went flying headfirst into the pavement. I try not to look at the eye, as I put the collar on his neck and get him down on the board. We get him in the back of the ambulance in no time flat. As soon as Shirley Lessard and Bruce Lincoln arrive in the second ambu-lance to take care of the girl, we take off for the hospital. A fire-fighter drives. When I go to put the nonrebreather on the patient's face, I have to look right down at the eye and bloody face. I shiver so hard, I heard the sound *hrrrurrr* escape from my mouth. I look away. I patch to the hospital to get the trauma room ready, then drill an IV in his left arm. Manny suctions blood from his airway and tries to calm him. We're out and rushing into the trauma room. Response time one minute. Scene time three minutes, transport two.

"High-speed motorcycle accident, no helmet, flew twenty feet, landed on his face. Massive facial trauma," I say. I point to his face. "No loss of consciousness. Alert and oriented. Vitals stable. Blood in his airway." I step back. I watch the faces of the doctors, nurses, and techs as they catch a glimpse of the eye. Their reactions are all similar to mine. They wince. Nasty.

They knock him out and try to tube him. The tube goes into the stomach and blood gushes out like an oil well. They try again. His whole face is fractured and unstable. The front part of his skull is basically free-floating on his face, top of skull, cheekbones, jaw, all broken off from the cranium. They have to trach him, cutting a hole in his throat to pass a tube into his lungs to protect his breathing. His head seems to swell in front of our eyes. They sit the eye back on his face where the socket once held it. It looks like a lifeless golf ball.

A couple nights later, I respond to an MVA on the highway. We come around a bend in the road and see it suddenly ahead. "Four-seven-one, holy shit," I say, into the mike. "We're out."

A tractor trailer is sprawled across the road. It looks like a dinosaur on its back with its neck broken. I see another car in the wreckage. I have to climb a cement embankment to get through the wreckage and to the driver, who the cop has said doesn't look good. I find the man crashed against the wall, his head caved in, his legs pinned. "What do you need?" my partner, Jack Early, asks.

"The monitor," I say.

I attach the leads. Flatline. I call him right there on the highway. Injury incompatible with life. I run my strip.

That night I have a dream. I am walking the countryside carrying a head in a black sack. I am trying to sell it, but I am not having much luck. I am on a hilltop among some apple trees when an attractive, well-dressed woman approaches me and says, "I hear you have a head for sale?"

"I do."

"May I see it?"

I take the head out and show it to her. "It's not a bad head," I say. "There is some dried blood and bruising about the nose and face, but it's still largely intact."

She studies it, saying nothing, pondering, wondering whether to invest in this head I have for sale. Finally she says, "Thanks for showing it to me. I'll get back to you on it."

"Okay," I say. "I'll be around."

I watch her walk off over the next hill. I put the head back in the bag and continue on my journey. I am just an ordinary man carrying some other guy's head.

# Nicki Joyner

I hear over the radio a basic crew being assigned a transfer—Nicki Joyner, going from the hospital to a nursing home. Nicki Joyner. A name I won't forget. I get on the phone and call dispatch. "Can we do this one?" I ask.

"Sure, if you want. It's just a basic run. No specials."

"We got a transfer," I say to Arthur, who has just put the stretcher back in the ambulance, after remaking the sheets and resupplying the rig.

"Oh, no," he says. "I just put the stretcher away."

"Nicki Joyner," I say. "Going to Mediplex. I requested it."

"Nicki Joyner," he says. He nods and says nothing more.

I feel trepidation going up in the elevator. The last time we saw her she was on our stretcher, not breathing. I had struggled with the tube. She'd coded, but I'd brought her back, though I have heard she has brain damage. I need to see her for myself, need to come to grips with it.

Outside the room, the nurse hands me the forms and says, she's been here for months. She runs down a list of complications: infections, impacted bowels, sepsis. She had an anoxic event, she says. Was in a nursing home for a while, then developed a fever that just wouldn't go away. I say nothing.

From the room, I can hear an aide talking to her as she changes her diaper. "You be all right now, pretty girl," the aide says.

I am hopeful that she can understand this. I walk in the room and see her now. She is in her thirties. Her hair is short and greasy, her face has a hundred or more whiteheads. I look at her eyes—they float in her head, but don't focus. Her eyes drift back and forth. She has a hole in her throat—a trach, through

157

which she gets oxygen from a mask. Although she is hemo-dynamically stable—a good blood pressure, pulse, and respirations on her own—she can't control her airway. If she were to choke on food, she wouldn't know it and would stop breathing. The trach lets her breathe without worry, but it is an enticement to infection.

"Does she respond at all?" I ask the nurse.

"She seem to move to voices sometimes, but no, dear, she's . . ."

Just then a man comes in the room. "What are they doing here?" he says. He is in his thirties; he goes right to her and strokes her head.

"They are taking her to Mediplex. Your family knows about it."

He nods, then whispers to her, "It's okay, Nicki girl. How are you today?"

He looks at us. I wonder if he was there, if he remembers us, but there is no look of recognition. "I didn't think she was going today," he says. "Can I get a ride with you?"

"Sure," Arthur says.

We move the stretcher up next to the bed and lower all the side rails. We take her foley bag and lay it on her feet, then grabbing the sheets, we prepare to move her.

"Okay, ma'am," I say, "We're just going to move you over to our bed."

"They're just going to move you, Nicki, honey," the man translates, running his hand over her forehead, then steps back to let us work.

We slide her over, then get her comfortable, putting another sheet over her foley bag. Her eyes move back and forth, seeing nothing.

The man comes down with us in the elevator. I want to ask him questions, but I don't know what to say, and I don't want to betray that we were the ones who responded, that if I had gotten the tube in time, none of this might have come to pass. I keep quiet.

He sits in the front, and I am alone in back with her. We go without lights and sirens because it is just a simple transfer.

I take her blood pressure and pulse and count her respirations, which I record. I shine a light into her eyes. No reaction at all. The pupils stay fixed. I look at her head. I think about how I tried to lift her tongue up and peer down into her cords. How they were hard to see, and then when I saw them, they were closed shut, and I couldn't pass the tube. How even when I tried to bag her, no air got through, and how it was only after her heart had stopped that I was able to finally get the tube in and get air back to her brain. Too late. Right here on this same stretcher, in this same ambulance, we'd fought and lost. If there was one call I could do over, this would be the one. If I'd tubed her and kept her brain alive, she'd have been out of the hospital and right now could be walking by on the street, or sitting on the stoop, drinking a beer with her boyfriend in the front seat, or maybe in the back bedroom with him, sweating and groaning.

I watch her eyes roll back and forth. I shine the light in them again. Nothing. Nothing.

I let out my breath and look up at the ceiling. I sit alone with my failure.

At the convalescent home we take her into her room, where the nurse knows all about her, having gotten a report on the telephone. Her boyfriend leans over the bed, talking to her, "Nicki, you're going to be okay, girl. You're going to be all right."

I watch him, my throat thickening.

He glances up. "Thank you," he says.

I keep looking at them. Then I walk over and put my hand on his shoulder. "Good luck," I say. The words seem to catch in my throat. "They'll take good care of her here."

He looks up at me. "Thank you, thanks again." He seems touched by it, touched that a faceless ambulance attendant would show concern for his plight, which is killing him, dragging his spirit down. "Thanks." He looks tired.

We leave the room. I take the front of the stretcher. "Don't you want the head end?" Art says.

I keep my back to him, not wanting him to see my eyes. "No,

it's okay," I say. I fight my emotion, and by the time we are out on the street, nothing betrays me.


# Body Count


We respond to a shooting. As we approach, an officer radios, "Just have the medic come in." I know what that means. It is a crime scene and the patient is probably dead. There are at least six police cars parked along the long driveway. I get out and bring the monitor and the in-house bag.

The officer meets me at the door. "He's been dead for a while. He looks all bled out. You'll see."

I walk through the house to the garage. In the garage a shirt-less man lies on his side in a fetal position against the door, a shotgun in his hands. He looks to be about thirty. There is a lake of red blood around his head that has grown out in grotesque inlets and coves and dried sticky. His skin color is translucent white. His bare feet are blue-purple where they touch the cold floor. From the kitchen I can hear a woman wailing. He is beyond any attempt at resuscitation. I look at my watch. "Presumed three-fifteen," I say.


We're called for an unknown on Hamilton Street. When we arrive an old man meets us on the street. "My wife, she's in the basement," he says.

"Which door?" I ask.

"Over there," he points. "I got up this morning."

He moves too slowly for us. There is a story he wants to tell us, but I am impatient to get to his wife.

I go through the door and down the basement steps. I see her then, a small tiny lady in her seventies, hanging from a wood beam, her neck bent, a milk carton by her feet. Her skin is cool. I put the monitor on, the leads on her hands and left ankle. She is asystolic. I look at my watch and mark the time.

The man is in the house now. Two officers have arrived, and I have shown them the body. "Is she all right?" the old man asks. "I got up this morning and she had a roll out for me, but she wasn't at the table."

"Come sit down over here," the officer says.

The two women are shaking and crying as we come through the door. In the bathroom lies a man, a bottle of nitro on the floor a few inches from his outstretched hand. He is cool, his jaw is stiff. Down a couple hours. They had gone out shopping.

"I'm sorry," I say, after I have run the required six-inch strip of asystole for documentation on my run form. I put the strip in my pocket. "I am sorry."

Tears run down their faces. They are Russian immigrants, in the country just a few months. Husband, brother, provider dead. They wail and tremble.

A truck driver, cold and stiff in the cab of his semi, a needle still in his hand. A sixty-year-old woman on the toilet, her mouth and eyes open staring at the ceiling, her jaw stiff. A young male, naked, lying facedown on the cold cement behind an abandoned building, his chest and head bludgeoned. Others. Many.

I look at my watch and record the times.

I run my strips.

# BURNOUT

*I just sit the rest of the way wondering what is happening to me.*

# Booking Off

To *book off* is to not come to work. People book off for many reasons—they are stressed out and need an unscheduled break, they have tickets to a baseball game, a crisis has arisen in their family, or they are too sick or hungover to get out of bed. I have never booked off. It helps that I work Tuesday, Wednesday, Thursday, seven in the morning to seven at night, and so I have a four-day weekend every week if I choose not to come in for overtime, which is plentiful. Still there have been days when I have thought seriously about booking off, when the last thing I wanted was to be at work. But a job like this, for me, anyway, requires discipline and routine. I fear that if I book off once, then it will be easier to book off the next time. Then I will start to slip, my whole manner will loosen, and I will stop caring. It may sound silly, but being dependable, being able to be counted on when my name is on the book to work, is part of my armor. It protects me from the dangers that are out there. It says nothing can rattle or break me. It makes me strong. It says I like my job even when it is weighing me down.

# Dead-icated

A new dispatch system is in place in Hartford. The standard practice has been for all cars to sign on with the Hartford Police dispatcher in the morning, giving the dispatcher the car number and the area of town they will be covering. HPD has now informed the company they want six "dedicated cars": two advanced life support (ALS) cars, and four basic life support (BLS) cars that go on line with them in the morning, stay under their control all day, and cannot be yanked to do transfers or calls in other towns. Sounds good to them, will make their lives easier. The problem is not apparent to them but soon becomes very apparent to us.

I am one of the on-line dedicated cars. I'm stationed in the north of town. The other five cars are all on calls. A call for a difficulty breathing comes in two blocks from Hartford Hospital—a five-minute response during rush hour. Two off-line paramedic cars are at Hartford Hospital. They are not allowed to respond. I clench the dashboard as Arthur hurls us across town, air horn slamming. The patient, who is cyanotic, his lungs filling with fluid, waits anxiously. I get an IV, put him on oxygen, and give 80 milligrams of Lasix, two nitros, and a Ventolin treatment. At Hartford Hospital, they intubate the patient.

I am an off-line paramedic sitting at Saint Francis, talking with Shawn Kinkade, another off-line paramedic, when the call goes out for chest pain on Homestead Avenue, two blocks away, and HPD dispatches a basic ambulance from Hartford to respond. We are not allowed to go to the call, even though the patient has chest pain and needs a paramedic who can arrive five

166

minutes earlier than the basic, who has only oxygen for the patient. "Can we head over that way?" I ask dispatch.

"No, I want you to take one out of Saint Fran radiology going back to Alexandria Manor." Shawn is dispatched to pick up Mrs. Greenberg at Mount Sinai dialysis. When I come down with our patient, we see the basic crew bringing the patient in with another BLS crew, CPR in progress. The patient is blue from the neck up, vomit around his mouth and on the stretcher. Sixty-two years old. No medic available.

"This is ridiculous," I say to Shawn later when I tell him the chest pain turned out to be a code. "I don't see how they can let this continue."

Shawn just shakes his head. He is dispirited. "Nobody cares," he says.

The world is turned upside down. It is a surreal system. Basics doing codes; medics doing transfers.

The company is reluctant to dedicate more medics because we need to be able to pull the medics off-line, if we have to meet contracts in other towns. If a 911 call goes off in Newington, we are contractually bound to send another paramedic car to Newington. If all the medics are dedicated to Hartford, they can't go to Newington or Windsor or West Hartford. So while the company is supposedly keeping us off-line to save us for the contracted towns because all the basic cars are now online, the medics end up doing the most basic nonemergency transfer calls.

The dispatching system is a disaster. Cars pass each other going lights and sirens to opposite ends of town. The Hartford Police Dispatch is dramatically understaffed. The lone dispatcher allocated to EMS is unable to interview 911 callers for any meaningful length of time; consequently we are sent priority one for a difficulty breathing that turns out to be a four-year-old boy who has had a runny nose for two weeks and his mom wants to take him to the doctor, or for a severe bleeding that turns out to be a twenty-four-year-old man who cut himself shaving and wants a Band-Aid. Often we are sent to calls and told by the caller on our arrival that they didn't want an ambulance, they just wanted the police. Some suspect HPD is using us to check out calls because all the police officers on duty are tied up on other calls. It is not uncommon for an EMS crew to be sent for a head injury or cut hand and walk in unaware to a full-blown assault in progress, and then to be unable to raise the police on the portable radio because the EMS dispatcher is on the phone taking another 911 call. Chris Carcia and Mike Carl call a "10-0," crew in distress, when a patient turns on them. Three ambulance crews respond before the first police officer can get there. Fortunately, Mike has taken the man down, and is pinning him, arm behind his back, face pressed against the carpet.

We are told our company has offered to take over all EMS dispatching for the city. From the company's point of view, it makes sense. Unlike the police dispatchers, our dispatchers are all medically trained, and having the ability to control our entire fleet—at times over twenty cars—rather than just the six dedicated cars, will improve response time and get paramedics to the calls where they are truly needed. HPD wants no part of the offer. They don't trust the company to watch over itself. While they need a way to hold us accountable, there has to be a better system. The company is leery of upsetting HPD because while we have the state designated Public Service Area (PSA), giving us the legal right to respond to all 911 calls, Hartford can attempt to take the designation from us, and the rumor is they want to give part of the town to another company with political connections. We can't afford to upset them, or so the story goes. One day there are no medics on-line. The company puts two Intermediate cars on to meet the ALS requirements. Intermediates, while called ALS, are only able to do IVs and insert a combi-tube in a nonbreathing patient, an airway adjunct not as effective as an endotracheal tube. They cannot give meds and do not even carry semiautomatic defibrillators.

Nobody thinks the system will last, but week after week it is still in place. At least the company, at the EMTs' prodding, abandons the Intermediates and replaces them with two medic cars. I get on-line once a week, while the rest of the days are a mix of nursing home emergencies, transfers, and an occasional

911 in a neighboring town or an intercept with a volunteer service. Some days are all transfers.

Arthur and I are sent to pick up Mrs. Greenberg at her home in an exclusive section of West Hartford. The maid meets us at the door and leads us down a hallway with gold-framed paintings and marble statues on teak tables. In the back library we find Mrs. Greenberg sitting in a wheelchair, reading a book, *Death and Suffering*. She has wrinkled skin and dark suspicious eyes. She is probably seventy.

"Who are you? You're new. I've never seen you before."

"Well," Arthur says, "I've worked here for seven years, my partner for three. We've never seen you before."

"Well, you're new to me. I don't like it when they send new people."

"Well, we go where we're sent," Arthur says. "We're not allowed to choose."

"You know how to get there?"

"Yes."

We lower the stretcher, move it next to the wheelchair.

"I'll get her arms, you get her legs," I say to Arthur.

"What are you doing?" she says. "That's not how the others do it."

"This is how we do it," I say.

I reach under her arms from the back and grasp her forearms, while Arthur holds her under her legs. We lift her up and over to the stretcher.

"Ow," she says. "You're hurting me. Ow! Stop."

She is already on our stretcher now.

"I'm very sorry," I say.

"You hurt me."

"I'm sorry. I didn't mean to. I don't like to hurt people. I try to avoid hurting people."

"Well, you hurt me. It still hurts."

"Like I said, I'm very sorry."

"I told you not to hurt me. I don't like new people."

"Ma'am. I have apologized three times, I don't know what else I can do."

"Make it stop hurting."

I nod and say nothing. Arthur laughs at me as we wheel her out of the house and carry her down the four front steps. I smile at Arthur as we load her into the ambulance, then I hold the door open for him to get in back with her. I'm driving.

All the way to the dialysis center, I hear her in the back. "He hurt me. He's so strong. I thought he was going to break my arm, that big terrible man, he hurt me." Arthur apologizes again and again. On the radio calls go out. Gunshot, asthma, chest pain. BLS units responding. All priority one. I turn off the HPD radio. I don't even want to hear it.

One day Arthur and I do eight transfers in a row without a break.

At two in the afternoon we clear Hartford dialysis, and Arthur asks on the radio, "Can we get a one-oh-three," meaning a lunch break.

"No, take one out of Hartford ER, going to Salmon Brook in Glastonbury, no specials, then you can get a bite."

Arthur starts to fume. I see his face turn red, he unleashes a stream of swear words, then grabs the mike, and says, "Yeah, maybe we can get a tray!" then slams the mike down.

He's angry, but I am laughing. And I will learn that all over the city, medics and their partners are rolling in their seats. "Did you hear what Arthur said? 'Maybe we can get a tray.'"

Busting our butts all day long and only being able to eat by begging a cafeteria tray of food from a nursing home kitchen. It kills me. "That was good, Arthur, 'Maybe we can get a tray.' That was funny. That was really funny."

"Fucking dispatch," Arthur says.

The next week we are sent to a nursing home in Bloomfield to take a nonverbal ninety-year-old patient with Alzheimer's and two broken legs to her doctor's office in Hartford. She is on oxygen, breathing about twenty-eight breaths a minute. She looks like she is about to expire. We get to the doctor's office, but they have no place to put her and no oxygen, so we have to wait there with her. They say they will try to hurry things along for us, and rather than make us wait in the waiting room with the other twenty patients, they let us wheel her into a small examining room, where we sit with her for two hours, reading magazines. I haven't brought the HPD portable, which is good because I would be getting annoyed at all the calls going out to basic units, all the cries for medics. I sit by the window, watch the rain pour down, and hear an ambulance wail past on the street below. I read a *Scientific American* about gamma rays from distant galaxies blowing up. I read a *Sports Illustrated* article about playground legends. Arthur reads a car magazine.

"Oh, my God," Arthur says.

"What?"

"Nothing, I just wanted to make sure she was still breathing."

I look at her. She is still plugging away.

I ask how the $O_2$ is.

"Another hour and we'll have to go get a spare tank."

Finally, we take her across the hall to X ray, where Arthur is recruited to wear an iron apron and hold the lady's legs while they take X rays.

I turned down the offer, volunteering Arthur because he already has his share of kids. "I'll be across the hall," I say.

"Four-seven-one," the company is calling on the portable.

"Four-seven-one."

"Four-seven-one, how are you doing?"

"We're in X ray now," I say cheerfully. "Art's wearing an iron apron, and holding the patient's leg in place."

"Okay," she says tiredly.

After the X rays are done, we wait another half an hour for the doctor to come in, which he does, bursting into the room, looking at the lady, and grunting to Arthur, who says hello. He examines her, then leaves the room.

"Charismatic guy," I say.

"Yeah, let's invite him to the pig roast," Arthur replies.

He comes back with a cast cutter, and Arthur and the nurse hold the lady's leg while he uses the saw to cut the cast open. He has a long tie that I keep hoping will get in the way and get sawed in half. He gets the cast off, then uses some bandage scissors to cut the cotton dressing inside. The woman has some nasty decubitus, pressure sores inside, which he wraps with more gauze. Then he puts on a soft splint.

He cuts some of the cast off the other leg, but leaves most of it on. He looks around for his bandage scissors but can't find them. Arthur offers him his trauma shears, which he takes again with just a grunt, then sets on the table when he is done.

He leaves the room again. I pick up the trauma shears and hand them to Arthur. "Thanks for lending them to me," I say.

"You're quite welcome, doctor. I'm happy to be of service."

I spot the bandage scissors on the chair, under the cast cutter, and I am thinking about swiping them or maybe just hiding them when the nurse comes back in to collect all the instruments. The doctor pops his head back in and says, "You can take her to the front window and they'll schedule a follow-up appointment."

Okay.

The receptionist asks how a month from today is.

Arthur looks at the lady on the stretcher. We both study her. "I don't know," Arthur says.

"She may have bridge that day," I say.

"Why don't you call the nursing home?" Arthur asks. "They keep her schedule."

"Have them call us," she says.

Arthur nods.

"Can I have one of these pens?" I ask, pointing to the cup of pens with the doctor's practice on it.

"Go ahead, and take one for a friend," another receptionist answers.

"I will," I say, handing one to Arthur. "For you."

A week later, the pen runs out of ink halfway through a run form.

I am talking with Debbie Haliscak and Greg Berryman about the new citywide EMS protocols. "We need one on houseplant care," I say.

"I always keep my trauma shears handy," Greg says, "for clipping the brown leaves before they spread disease."

"What do you water them with, normal saline or lactated ringers?"

"Normal saline. The lactate makes the leaves droop."

I tell him about my method of using the nebulizer we use for asthmatics to moisten the leaves.

"I'll have to try that. . . . How about epi?" he asks.

"Do not give epi to Venus's-flytraps," I say. "I read on the Internet that a medic in New York state lost a finger to a combative plant."

"Cardiology is hard, but plant care is much more demanding," Greg says.

"What breaks my heart," I say, "is the plant care in some of the nursing homes we go into. Hellholes, I tell you."

Just then my radio calls. They send us to Windham, a forty-minute ride out of town. A basic transfer. As we hit the outskirts of town, I hear two chest pains go out to basic units.


# Stress


Car 884 is dispatched to an unknown on Hampton Street. A moment later we're told to head to New Britain General Hospital for a transfer. As soon as we get on the ramp to I-84 West we hear our company dispatcher asking, "eight-eight-four, are you all right?" There is static. "What's going on?" Simultaneously, HPD dispatches another car. "We have a ten-ten, ambulance rollover."

Both Arthur and I want to spin around and race to the scene, but we're on another call, plus every other ambulance is asking to head that way. Dispatch tells cars to stay clear. "We have one ambulance headed to the scene and two supervisors in eight-four-zero rushing to back them up." Rick Ortyl and Shannon

Pratt are in 884. I can hear Shannon through the static saying, "We're okay," but her voice sounds shaken. The fire department is dispatched for extrication.

We're quiet as we head away from the city, listening, waiting.

One ambulance goes to Hartford on a priority two, the other on a priority three.

When we get to New Britain, we call the office to ask for an update. Information is sketchy, but Rick and Shannon were both alert and talking at the scene. Shannon may have a hand and shoulder injury. Rick will probably be okay; he is just banged up.

Later we get the story. As they were going lights and sirens through the intersection of Chapel and High, a car that did not yield clipped them in the back by the passenger side and sent them over on their side. Rick fell down onto Shannon. The fire department had to take out the front window to get them out. In the article in the paper the next day, the police department will deny sending the ambulance on a priority. But unknowns are *always* priority two. Always go lights and sirens. Often HPD dispatches a call without giving a priority, but we go based on what it is. A shooting you go priority one. Same with chest pain. A drunk you go on a three.

Arthur is always mad when they don't give a priority, and I'll say, "It's an asthma, go on a two."

"But they're *supposed* to give a priority," he'll say. He'll call back and ask for a priority, and they'll say priority two. To me it's a waste of time, but he says if they don't give you a priority you're in trouble if you get in an accident.

"Yeah, right," I'll say, "If they dispatch us to a baby not breathing and don't give a priority, we're in trouble if we don't go on one. Common sense."

"They're supposed to give a priority," he'll say. Well, here's a case where he is right. The article in the paper makes the "ambulance drivers" look at fault.

Accidents are common in this business. They tell you if are in an accident and it's your fault, it's your fault. And they tell you if you get in an accident and it's not your fault, it's still your fault. All of our ambulances have a sign on the front dashboard that says we are required to come to complete stops at all red lights, intersections, and yield signs when using our lights and sirens. It's a good risk-management practice, but try stopping at thirty deserted intersections when you are going priority one for a child not breathing. In the various towns we respond to, we have contracted response times. The company is fined if we don't make the times.

At Saint Francis, I'm writing up my paperwork for the previous call and Arthur is resupplying the ambulance when we get called out to do a call deep into West Hartford for a chest pain. The dispatcher keeps coming over the radio to ask us how we're doing. "Just fine," Arthur says.

"I mean where are you?" the dispatcher says.

"Albany Avenue. We're doing our best."

When we get back to the office that night, a supervisor wants to know which of us was driving. Someone in management saw our car blow through a yellow light at a high rate of speed and was quite upset. "Let him come down here and tell us that to our face," I say, suddenly upset. "You haul us out of the hospital, send us deep into West Hartford for a chest pain, hound our butts all the way to the call—Where are you? Where are you? Howya doing? How far out?—worried about the response time, and you expect us to come to a complete stop at every intersection. Come on. Let him come down here and say it to our faces."

"I'm just passing on the complaint," the supervisor says.

Arthur is unconcerned about it. It is the last day of our rotation. "Time for me to get naked," he says, running his card through the punch clock.

# Meat in the Seat

With the company about to be bought by a large national company, we are all concerned about what may happen. In non-union companies bought by the corporation, the company has come in, fired everyone, then rehired whomever they wanted, often at lower wages. I have been reading stories from across the nation on an on-line EMS bulletin board. Paramedics who worked two twenty-four-hour shifts a week at sixteen dollars per hour, and worked part-time jobs on their days off are fired and offered new jobs working five eight-hour shifts at twelve dollars per hour, working three days on, a day off, two days on, a day off.

We are all worried. Some talk of finding work elsewhere. The problem is that there are few other places to work. The new company has also bought up much of our competition. They dominate the market.

We take a wait-and-see approach. Some of the things the new company is talking about sound good. They plan to put a paramedic in each car, which would be great for patient care. During my paramedic class I rode with an ambulance service before and then after it was bought by the company, and I have to say, the new company cleaned the place up, instituted a dispatch system that improved response, and thoroughly professionalized the operation. I hope that whatever changes they institute here will be for the better.

I talk to an employee who is worried he will lose his management job in the new company. "You don't have to worry about your job as a medic," he says to me. "They are always looking for meat in the seat."

# Snowstorm

We're in Bellevue Square in the middle of a blizzard. The access road to the public housing project has been plowed only once, and by a plow not much bigger than our ambulance. In the back we've got a guy who had surgery on his jaw a few days ago; he has run out of his medication so he called 911 for a ride to the hospital. The access road turns to the left. I shout hold on, because I don't think the road is wide enough to make the turn. I gun the engine, hoping the speed will get us through, but the wheels catch in the snowbank and the back spins out. We're stuck. I get out and look at the ambulance. It's cold and the snow is still coming down. We're backed up with calls all over the city. My partner tries to push, but we can't quite break free. I don't want to call dispatch. This would be the second time this winter I've gotten stuck at the same location. The door opens up, and our patient steps out. My partner and I look at each other. The patient looks at the wheel and shakes his head. He swears.

"You want to help push?" I say.

He shakes his head but puts his shoulder to the back corner.

I get in the front and hit the gas as they rock the rig back and forth. It breaks free, fishtails a moment, then finds purchase on the road. They get in back, patient and EMT, and we continue on to the hospital.

# Priorities

I am on line working with Kelly Tierney. We are parked by the graduate center just off Main Street. The police dispatcher gives us a call for an assault on Standish, way down off Wethersfield Avenue. Priority three. Two minutes later, the police dispatcher gives a priority one unresponsive call at the graduate center to 903, a basic car just coming on line. I ask Kathy Poulin, our company dispatcher, if she wants us to divert, switch calls with 903. "You can try the police," she says. "I was going to suggest that but their dispatcher hung up on me." The police dispatcher on duty is the only one who continually gives us a hard time. While many of the dispatchers there do an excellent job, this particular woman has no business being in her line of work.

"HPD, four-seven-one," I say. "We're at Main and Gold. Would you like us to divert to the graduate center?"

"No," she says emphatically.

"Just thought I'd suggest it," I say. "We're only a couple blocks away."

"So much for patient care," Kelly says. "She's too lazy to switch calls on the board."

Five minutes later we call out on Standish. A man under arrest by HPD has a cut finger. He is HIV-positive. The cops don't have anything to clean his hands with, so we take some saline and sterile dressings and start to clean the cut and the blood off his hands. On the radio we finally hear 903 put out. A few minutes later, they come on the radio screaming for a paramedic. They have to call four-seven-two out of Saint Francis to respond. They are just arriving on scene when we clear our call.

"Nobody cares," Kelly says. "It's as simple as that."

Another ten minutes later, 903 with the 472 medic leave on a priority to Hartford Hospital.

A forty-year-old Hartford man suddenly stops breathing while at the dinner table. No paramedic crew is available. When the basic unit arrives, he is not breathing. They try to ventilate him with the ambu-bag. They get some air in but not enough to fully expand his chest. He is now in full cardiac arrest. They do CPR. When the man is brought into the hospital, the doctor goes into his mouth with the laryngoscope to intubate and sees a giant piece of meat wedged deep in the windpipe. Using his Magill forceps, he removes the meat. The airway now clear, he intubates the man and works feverishly with the hospital staff to restore a heart rhythm. The man doesn't make it. Forty years old. Choked on a piece of meat. Too deep in his airway for the Heimlich manuever to work. A paramedic with a laryngoscope and Magill forceps—standard paramedic equipment, not issued to basics—responding to the 911 call could have saved his life on the spot. He might not have even needed to go to the hospital. But where were the paramedics? Doing transfers. Doing B.S. An avoidable death. A system failure. A system that everyone knew was broken. Hartford police department. The company. Medical control. Me.

# Mean Streak

Priority one. Bus accident involving children in the parking lot of a high school.

"It's bullshit, I know it's bullshit," I say. "What kind of accident can you have in the parking lot?"

"Somebody could get backed over," Art says.

I'm thinking in my gut he might be right. I feel it's bullshit, but you never really know.

Another car responds with us.

We're just down the street when the PD dispatcher radios, "Slow it down, minor injury."

When we arrive, the cop tells us there is only one person hurt, an eighteen-year-old kid lying on the ground outside the bus with a Walkman on. A couple of his friends are standing over him, laughing. The buses barely touched, the cop says, this kid walked off the bus, lay down, said his back and neck hurt. It's bullshit, the cop says.

Greg Berryman, the other medic, and I walk over to the kid. The kid is wearing a Tommy Hilfiger shirt, baggy jeans, and a pair of Air Jordans. Styling. Jiggy.

"What's the matter, kid?"

"I hurt all over," he says. "The buses collided, and I banged my head." He tries to suppress a giggle.

"Okay," I say. "We're going to have to C-spine you. That means putting a collar on your neck and strapping you to a board. Are you sure you're hurt?"

"Yeah, I'm hurt. Look at them laughing at me. Man, I'm hurt. All over. Neck, back. Nearly busted my head."

Okay.

We C-spine him. The whole routine. Heavy tape over the eyebrows. Get him in the back of the ambulance.

I take his blood pressure. I squeeze the balloon hard, pumping it up: 200, 300, around again to 100, 200. I look at his hand now. It is slowly turning white. I press against his nail beds. His capillary refill is delayed. "You're going to need an IV," I say. "Capillary refill delayed. That's a bad sign."

"What?" the guy says.

"Large-bore IV," Greg says. "Maybe dual fourteens."

"Definitely. Could be eternal bleeding."

"Pupil check," Greg says. I glance at him and see he has the spotlight in his hands. This is the spotlight that can burn a hole in the floor of the ambulance, if accidentally left on. "Constricted," Greg says, without shining it in his eyes; if he did, it would leave the boy seeing spots for weeks.

"Why are you all laughing?" the kid says.

"You need laughter in this job to mask the horrible things we see. You're injured. We're going to need to do an IV if there is any chance at all."

"What?"

"No need to be too concerned. Yet."

"I just hurt; I ain't sick."

"Cut his clothes," I say.

"What are you doing? That's my shirt."

"You're hurt, we've got to expose you fully to make sure we don't miss anything. It's protocol. It's our job."

"Oh, man."

We make quick work of the Hilfiger jacket and jeans. Cut the laces of the sneakers.

"Looks okay, no obvious deformities. I guess we can take it on a three."

"I can't believe you cut my clothes, man. Who's gonna pay for that?"

I shrug.

"Man."

"How's your neck?"

"Huh?"


At the hospital, we put him in the back hall and tell him not to move until he is cleared. He protests, but I tell him any insurance claim is void if he gets up. But he has to take a leak, he says. I tell him I'll bring him a urinal.

I see the nurse and give the report. Complete bullshit, I say. I tell her he needs to take a leak. "I'll bring him the urinal," I say. I know she is busy.

"Man, I got to pee," I hear him say as I walk past. "I ain't kidding. You going to get me something so I can pee." I keep walking on down the hall and out the door.

"You know, buried beneath all the nice guy stuff you really

do have a mean streak in you," Arthur says when I get in the
ambulance.

"Teach him to fuck with the system." I am still angry.

# Roles

A crew is dispatched for a seizure. Just as they turn the corner,
they are canceled; the police have transported. That night
on the news the story makes the cops look like heroes for
"saving the baby's life." The baby, by the way, is released from
the hospital hours after being brought there. The diagnosis—a
febrile seizure—is a common, rarely life-threatening event for
babies. A week later, on TV, the cops are given a plaque by the
baby's mother and a commendation by the department. No one
asks the hospital for their opinion of the officers' actions—that
indeed if the child truly weren't breathing, they endangered
him by driving him to the hospital, taking it away from the immediate lifesaving care of the paramedics who could put a tube
into the child's trachea and breathe air back into his lungs,
keeping his brain cells alive.

A number of years earlier, an EMT was called to the scene of
a shooting. He arrived to see the getaway car pull away. To the
horror and dismay of his coworkers, he chased after the car and
radioed its location and description to the police. He received a
commendation from the state's attorney. Meanwhile medical
control wanted to yank his certification for abandoning the
scene before doing his job: checking to see if anyone was hurt.
And his coworkers, who have to treat the lawful and the un-
lawful equally and without judgment, faced the threat of gang
payback.

In both cases, the people flagrantly disregard their duty and possibly endanger patients. In both cases they get awards.


# State Card


The call is for chest pain. A man will be standing at the corner of Collins and Woodland. We're covering area three—Saint Francis. We're parked in the ER lot at the corner of Collins and Woodland. I see a guy come out of the waiting room and walk over to the corner. We pull up. I look at him through the passenger window. He motions for me to roll the window down. I do.

"I called for the ambulance," he says. "I got chest pain. For two weeks. Hurts like hell when I breathe." He has alcohol on his breath.

"The hospital's right there," I say. I point to the ER door.

"Take me to Hartford Hospital. I got no use for Saint Francis. I'm tired of waiting. I been waiting there for four hours. They said it's my fault I was sleeping when they called my name. They could of had the courtesy—they could of had the courtesy to wake a brother up now, couldn't they? Ain't my fault I been waiting so goddamned long. My chest is killing me, man. Coughing up green shit all damn day long. Here's my card." He holds out his state medical card. Holds it like it is cab fare, which it is.

"Get in," I say.

When we get to Hartford, they put him in their waiting room.

# Quit

A paramedic I really respect comes into St. Francis with a patient from a car accident, a young woman who is actively seizing. He is upset because the extrication took too long and he couldn't get a line. The young woman is badly injured, and she needed Valium to stop the seizing. He is exhausted, spent. There is blood on his shirt, his hair is mussed. He walks back from the trauma room, looking defeated. Half an hour later, I see him coming down the hall from upstairs, carrying three balloons and a plant, pushing the stretcher on which a woman sits. Her daughter says to him, "Be extra careful with her, her back is sore." He just nods, an unhappy look on his face.

I am talking to his partner a few weeks later, and I say how I think he is one of the medics I really look up to. "You haven't been riding with him the last couple months," she says. "He's burnt."

Another medic I respect quits unexpectedly. I meet him for a beer one night and he tells me why he couldn't go on. "I get called for an unknown. I find the lady—forty years old—lying in bed in her underwear. Nothing's wrong with her other than her wrist's sore. She says she's not ready to go yet. She has to call her sister to come watch her kids, and she's got to get dressed, and she can't find her medical card. I said, what do you mean you're not ready to go. You called nine-one-one. You called nine-one-one! I came here lights and sirens, and you're not ready to go!" He shakes his head in disbelief. "For this I spent five years of my life, working all kinds of bad hours." He drinks his beer. "I quit. I quit a long time ago."

# Shit Rising

The woman is four hundred pounds, lying on the kitchen floor, with brown puke flowing out of her mouth like lava. The woman is in cardiac arrest. She is not breathing and has no pulse. Her son is doing chest compressions and mouth-to-mouth ventilations on her. I try not to look at the puke stains on his face and shirt. I tell Bob Anderson to run down and get the suction. She is going to be hard enough to tube, having no neck. I tear her dress open. Her breasts are like two giant watermelons. I apply the monitor to her and she is asystole. Flatline. The family last saw her up fifteen minutes ago. She is only forty-nine, but at her size, she is not a healthy woman. High blood pressure, diabetes, they say. I am thinking about all the puke that is going to be in her throat when I open it up. That and how hard she is going to be to tube and how she looks like she doesn't have a visible vein on her, much less a jugular in her nonexistent neck. With all the puke in her mouth, I cannot get any air in with the ambu-bag, even with an oral airway. Bob is back quickly with the suction. I lay down on my belly and fight not to retch. I open her mouth, and the puke erupts again, dribbling down her eyes and ears and chin, puddling at the base of her head. I put a pillow under her back and stick the steel blade in, sweeping her tongue aside. It is like I am looking into the first floor of a house flooded up to the ceiling by a muddy river. I stick the suction in and listen to its slurpy whir. The water level slowly lowers and I can finally see the white vocal cords. I pull the suction out and grab for my tube, but the puke water level rises back to the ceiling, obscuring my view. I suction, the water goes down to reveal the cords, but again as

**185**

soon as I remove it, the crappy water rises back up. "I can't believe all this puke," I say aloud. "I can't see a fucking thing." No matter how much I suction, the shit keeps rising back to the top. Suction. Rise. Suction. Rise. I say screw it, I take the tube and jab right where I know the cords are. I feel the tube pass through. I inflate the balloon, check my lung and stomach sounds. More on the right than the left. Nothing over the stomach. I pull back on the tube a little till I hear the sounds equal on the left, then secure the tube. We fire drugs down the tube. Epi. Atropine. But the woman stays flatline. We try pacing—applying a steady electrical beat to the heart—but get no response. More epi. Atropine. Still nothing. We slide a board under her and secure her with three belts, still doing CPR. I look over my shoulder and see several family members watching us openmouthed, including two girls about eight or nine years old. "Why don't you take them into the other room?" Missy Young says. She and Chaz Milner have arrived to assist us.

"That's their grandmother," someone says.

"Please. We're going to need room to get by."

I didn't even know they were standing there. I should have been watching my language. Bob is trying to move the stretcher over, but the family won't get out of the way. "Please," he says.

I take the head end of the board and try to lift, but she is so top-heavy, I can't even budge it. Bob has to grab the side and help me. We stumble backward and finally get the board on the stretcher. A family member trying to help nearly topples me off balance.

I think if they wanted to help, they could have kept the fried chicken and pork chops out of her hands. This thought, at least, I keep to myself.

We wheel her down the hall in the low position. I realize her breasts are still exposed, but there isn't a sheet handy, and besides, she really isn't even a *she* to me anymore. She is a corpse. Flat on the monitor. Squeeze the ambu-bag. Compress the chest. If the family hadn't all been there, I might have called medical control and asked permission to call her dead right there on the floor. There is no bringing her back.

Now comes the fun part. The stairs or the elevator. "I'm not taking the stairs," I say.

"She won't fit in the elevator," Chaz says.

"Yes, she will."

The elevator door opens, and I have Bob help me lift. We lift the stretcher up so it is standing on end, the woman facing the back of the elevator door, standing for the last time. It fits perfectly. I hit first floor. "See you down there," I say.

The ride doesn't take long. I stand there looking at the stretcher and the obese dead woman strapped to it. I am as out of breath as if I've been moving a piano. And that's what it feels like to me. A moving job. I know that is not right. That is not what I should feel, but it is how I feel. I look at my pants and my shirt and see puke on them. I am damp with sweat. I am tired. I keep thinking, Why did you eat all that bacon and sausage and fried food? Couldn't you get a salad or go out for a jog instead of stuffing your fat face? Then I think about the dead woman sharing the elevator with me, standing for the very last time, her feet on the floor, her belly, which is most of her, pressed against the wall of the elevator. Have some respect.

The elevator hits the ground level, and we lower her out, continue our CPR out to the ambulance, where it takes four of us to lift her in back, then we continue on down the street to the hospital. Ventilate. Compress. Flatline.

They call her dead in the cardiac room.

# Burnout

I'm working overtime in the city and it has been a busy, hot day. I've done two room-one traumas, including a man out of his mind on cocaine who leapt out of a third-floor window and broke both his legs—nasty bilateral open tib/fib and foot fractures. It took four cops and me to wrestle him onto our stretcher. It was impossible for us to properly immobilize him to protect his spine. The cops had to handcuff him to the stretcher. Two cops rode with me in the back; I was unable to do anything for him. With his face he fought the oxygen mask that I tried to press against him. He spat and cursed. He was completely out of his mind.

Now we're sent for a pedestrian struck north on Main Street. There is a huge crowd in the street, always the sign of something bad. People are shouting, pushing each other. A woman lies in the middle of the road. Someone says she was struck by a car going forty and thrown twenty feet. She has a small hematoma on her head and pain in her ribs and says she hurts all over. I tell my partner, "Let's just get her out of here." We get her on the board and head to Saint Francis on a priority. I give a patch and ask for the trauma room. Then I spike a bag and put a tourniquet on her arm. "What are you doing?" she screams. "I ain't getting no needle. You ain't giving me no needle."

"Hold still," I say. "This won't hurt much and it will be over before you know it."

She swings her arm wildly. "No, no, I hate needles. You ain't giving me no needle."

"Listen," I say. "You need this. Hold still."

"I'm getting out of here. You stop the ambulance and let me out."

I lie to her. "If you don't get this needle, you could die."

"I don't care, I don't care." She sits up straight, breaking loose from her immobilization.

She is screaming at me. It is sweltering hot in the back.

"What the fuck is wrong with you? You want to die? You want me to help you or not?"

"Just don't give me a needle. I hate needles. Please let me out of here, I want to go home."

I am thinking, Here I am dripping with sweat, I've called for the trauma room for a patient who I am thinking now is not nearly as hurt as I thought. I don't have her C-spined, she's not on oxygen, and I don't have an IV. What am I doing busting my butt for these people who don't care?

"Why are you yelling at me?" she says, crying. "Why are you yelling at me?"

"I'm sorry," I say. "It's because I want to help you."

"Just don't give me no needle, please don't give me no needle."

I just sit the rest of the way wondering what is happening to me.

# Shame

It is six at night, the end of another long day. We're sent crosstown for a difficulty breathing postsurgery. Priority one. Franklin Avenue, second floor.

We pull up outside the address. It is a nice three-story apartment house. A large man in a New England Patriots T-shirt comes down the stairs and waves at us. "I bet it's an old lady," I say to Arthur as I reach for a pair of gloves. I step out of the ambulance. I fasten the HPD radio to my belt. I stuff the gloves in my pocket. Then I open the side doors, and take out the heart monitor and the heavy blue house bag. Arthur has gone around to the back to pull out the stretcher. "Let's just see what we have," I say.

We go through the front gate, then up the stairs to the porch, where the man, who is sweating heavily, stands anxiously. "I guess you're not like they are on TV."

"How's that?" I say.

"You're moving so slow. My son's having trouble breathing." He starts up the stairs, and I climb up behind him. It is a young man, which means it is likely to be B.S., but he seems concerned so maybe it is real. Then I start thinking, I am not going to let him talk to me and put me down like that. I've been busting my butt all goddamned day. You can't go running up every set of stairs, lugging this equipment. As we move into the apartment now, through a cluttered living room to the back hall, I finally let my frustration out. "I can't run with all this crap on the floor."

The man stops at the hallway entrance and looks back at me, and for a moment, I am thinking, Oh, I did it now. He's going to deck me. "You weren't even up here when you pulled in, so you didn't know there was anything on the floor and still you're moving slow. Please, my son." He turns and heads down the hall.

I follow.

"In here," he says.

On the bed there is a large young man in athletic shorts and T-shirt, lying on the bed, gasping. A pretty young woman sits on the bed comforting him.

"Excuse me, please," I say.

She is slow to get out of my way, and I think of commenting, but I hold my tongue, angry at myself for losing my temper.

I look at the boy. His eyes are closed and when I ask him what hurts, his lips move in a whisper that is inaudible. With his hand, he motions toward his chest. I put him on the pulse oximeter, then feel his pulse. His rate is regular, strong. The oxygen saturation reads 100 percent.

"He got out of surgery this afternoon and now he can't breathe," the man says.

"Well, he's getting oxygen just fine," I say. "One hundred percent. That's better than I'm doing." I listen to his lung sounds on both sides. Nice and clear. "Where does it hurt?"

Again, he does his inaudible mumble.

"What kind of surgery did he have?"

"A hernia operation. They knocked him out and had him on a ventilator."

I take his blood pressure: 110/70. Again fine. This is a healthy nineteen-year-old, who is probably just feeling nauseated from his surgery, playing his dad and his girlfriend for sympathy.

"He's okay," I say. "This is not life threatening."

"He's my boy. I'm his father and his mother, too. I didn't know what to do."

"Look, I'm sorry I snapped at you," I say. "We've had a long day. They train us not to run. If we fall and hurt ourselves carrying this gear, or miss something in the scene, then we're no good to anyone. I shouldn't have snapped. I was tired. It was unprofessional. I'm sorry."

"That's okay," he says. "I understand. It was just my boy wasn't breathing right."

"I understand. What hospital do you want to go to?"

"Hartford Hospital. It's where he had the surgery."

"Okay, let's go. Get up," I say to the boy.

"I don't think he can walk," the father says.

"He didn't have the operation on his legs," Arthur says. "He ought to be able to walk."

"He's too big to carry," I say. "It's safer for him to walk."

We each grab an arm and start pulling him up. He resists a bit, but we grab under his arms and get him up. He walks with his eyes closed, leaning on me.

Arthur takes the gear downstairs and I walk with the boy. His father also holds his arm. As we reach the top of the stairs, he starts to lean harder on me. I stand in front of him, so he won't fall down the stairs. At the bottom of the stairs, the boy starts to puke. His father and I hold him. He gives his weight up to us, so that if I drop him, he will fall. The puke, just watery juice, splashes by my boots. Art is at the car, his back turned to us, putting the gear in and getting the stretcher out and making it.

"Arthur," I call.

He doesn't turn. It is taking all my strength to hold the kid up.

"Arthur."

"He can't go on," the father says.

"He's okay," I say. "He's just nauseated from the surgery. . . . Arthur!"

Arthur finally turns and sees me holding the kid at the top of the outside stairs.

"Bring the stretcher over, please."

He gets the stretcher over; the boy takes the last four steps, then we set him on it. We lift him into the back of the ambulance. He must weight two hundred and forty pounds.

"We're not going to go lights and sirens," I say to the father, "and we're going to do a couple things in the back first."

I tell Arthur to spike a bag. I put a tourniquet around the boy's arm. He doesn't really need an IV, in my opinion, but his complaint, chest pain and difficulty breathing, coupled with the vomiting, qualify for one under the protocols. I am giving it to him for those reasons, and because of house rules. You can't walk on your own, you get an IV. I take out a fourteen—the biggest size we carry. I unwrap it, and though his eyes are closed, he jerks awake, and pulls his arm back. Spying on me, I think.

"Hold still," I say. "You need an IV. It's just a little poke."

I jab the vein. Blood flashes back. I draw four tubes of blood, then attach the IV. I tell Art we're all set to go. En route I put him on the monitor, give him a little oxygen.

"Feeling better?" I ask.

He nods.

In triage, while I am telling the story to the nurse, a clerk

comes over and asks the name of our patient. She says his father is here. They let him in.

"This is the father," I tell the nurse.

"And his mother, too," the man says. "And I got another boy
at home."

"Good for you," Arthur says. "He's a fine-looking boy. You
must be doing a good job with them."

"I'm doing my best. They are good boys." To the nurse, the
father says, "He had me worried, but he's looking better now.
These young men made him better." He nods to us. "Thank
you."

I smile back, but behind it, I feel shame. It was a B.S. call—
the kid was just nauseated from his surgery—but that doesn't
give me the right to act like I did.

I am better than this.


# Flat Line


I recognize what is going on. It is not the first time I have felt
this way. It is an occupational hazard. It comes in waves.
Sometimes it hovers like a fog, a haze. I try working through it.
Maybe a good call will change it. But the more I work, the
worse it grows. I try taking time off. Getting out of town.
Maybe a day at the beach, feeling the sun burn my face,
riding the Atlantic ocean saltwater waves, drinking beer and
eating clams into the night, looking at the stars and the moon,
feeling the sea breeze, nestling in tight with my girlfriend.

But it stays longer this time. I get out here and it is all
bullshit. I stop reading the educational journals. Stop carrying
my medical books. Stop following up on patients. Even the
good calls don't excite me. I go through them like a robot,

doing my job, but not caring, sometimes not even introducing myself. No longer face to face. It's vein to vein. Run form to run form. Just barely legible scribble on the page, followed by my signature on the bottom. A *P* followed by a *C* that turns into a long flat line.

# SHAMAN

*Will I be a good teacher? Will I be someone to look up to? . . . Will I soar above the city or will I crash in flames?*

# Reason

I talk to Debbie Haliscak, the EMS Coordinator at Saint Francis. "Debbie, I yelled at this lady the other day. I just lost it."

"You, yelling at a patient? I don't believe it."

"I just snapped. And it isn't the first time." I tell her how I am feeling, how it seems that what I do doesn't really matter. Driving priority one all the time, for what? Cut fingers, hyperventilation, bullshit. When I do use my paramedic skills, it is nothing that another paramedic couldn't do, but most of the time these days I am just a taxi service. And the system we have now doesn't even recognize my value. A transfer comes in and it doesn't matter if I am a medic or not, I get sent. Dialysis, basic transfer, even long-distance, out-of-town trips. It makes no sense. Basics doing codes while I am carrying flowers and balloons. And when I am on line, HPD doesn't care whether I'm a medic or not. "I'm in a deep rut," I say. "I keep waiting for it to change. But I can't get out of it. It's affecting me. I'm worried I'm going to stop caring. I can see it happening."

She listens. She has heard what I am expressing before. It's a symptom of the job. Common. She knows I will be back, excited to tell her about some great call. Or just as easily, one morning I will walk in and tell her I am leaving the field. Done. Nothing would surprise her.

"And to make matters worse," I say. "I hear the governor and health commissioner are cutting all the EMS programs in the state. All the work I put in to building it up when I worked for the governor, and nothing is going to be left. It's like, why have I even bothered to make an appearance on the planet. They don't care about paramedics on the street, and they don't care about EMS in the state."

"You and I have talked about paramedic power before. You don't get together and speak up, it's not going to happen."

Just then, my radio goes off. A drunk at the corner of Albany and Vine. I just shake my head. I am tired and don't feel like taking on the world, much less giving a ride to a drunk.

# Keep Hope Alive

I am standing outside Hartford Hospital restocking my ambulance when Cressy Goodwin comes by. Cressy is an expert in mass casualty events and a longtime EMS activist in Connecticut.

"I hear you're getting involved in trying to stop these cuts," he says.

"Well, not exactly." He is talking about cuts in the state budget for EMS. All that I have done is tell an old friend at the state Office of Emergency Medical Services (OEMS) that I would think about writing a letter to the editor, and maybe posting a sign at the hospitals to alert people to the cuts. Neither of which have I done, though nearly two weeks have passed since I spoke with my friend.

"There's a lot of people out there angry about this," he says. "Do you have an e-mail address?"

I give it to him hesitantly.

A few days later I get a phone call from Betty Morris, who is the regional coordinator for the North Central EMS Region. She asks my opinion on EMS leaders requesting a meeting with the governor.

"The hell with just meeting with the governor," I say. "You

have to march on the capitol." After our phone conversation, I make the mistake of putting my thoughts in writing and e-mailing them to her in a memo titled "Battle Plan," which details a multipronged approach of letter-writing, phone calls, and individual and organizational protests culminating in a rally at the state capitol.

Before a week has passed my plan has been circulated across the state and over the Internet.

Initially there seems to be genuine enthusiasm. My dormant political juices suddenly stirring, I write a flyer, which I post at hospitals in the area. I send a modified version to the *Hartford Courant* as a letter to the editor.

### Stand up for EMS!

We risk our lives and health to help those in need. The pay isn't good, and many volunteer for nothing. The work is tough, but it is honest, and our presence makes a difference in the world. The tone goes off, they call our number, and we go.

Most of us are too busy trying to support our families to pay much attention to what happens at the State Capitol. **The news, snuck into the new state budget, isn't good, and unless we speak up, it will only get worse.**

Since 1995, **the state's commitment to EMS has been rapidly abandoned.** Proposals for increased EMS funding have been squashed. Regional Council budgets cut. Support for the state conference ended. Ideas of the EMS Advisory Board ignored. OEMS has been demoted within the Health Department. **Positions have been slashed.** The Deputy OEMS Director and Head of Education eliminated. The EMS data specialist transferred. Now the state OEMS director and the head of EMS regulation are having their jobs axed. **The law requiring an EMS director is being skirted by pinning the title on an overburdened Health Bureau Chief with no EMS experience.** And a federal EMS assessment team, whose 1991 report on Connecticut EMS led to significant gains (the reestablishment of an EMS advisory committee with strong medical input, hiring an EMS director after a nationwide search, the establishment of the statewide trauma network, and a move toward statewide protocols) has been *disinvited* from their scheduled April 1997 review.

What does this mean for us on the street and our patients? It means **Connecticut EMS will fall further behind national standards.** The effort to bring all EMS systems up to top medical standards will cease. Federal funding lost. Curtailed support for volunteer services. **PSAs possibly abolished. EMS policy set by people with no EMS background.** Lengthy delays at the state office. Investigations of EMTs and paramedics conducted by people who have never been in the field. **We will be a laughingstock for other states. And we—EMS—will have no voice for our issues and concerns at a time when health care delivery is being revolutionized.**

**Don't let them disrespect us any longer.** Call Governor Rowland and your state Representatives today. **Tell them EMS—what we do—is important.** Tell them to reverse the EMS cuts. And tell them you will not forget how they stand on this issue.

Posting the flyer, I feel like Tom Paine, the revolutionary pamphleteer. I give ambulance crews copies of it to post in their bays, and I spend a day at home folding, stuffing, licking, and stamping 269 envelopes, mailing a copy to each EMS service— volunteer, commercial, first responder—in the state. Cressy sends the flyer out over the Internet, and soon it is posted in the emergency department of hospitals throughout the state.

"People are excited," Cressy tells me. "There's a groundswell out there."

Others set a date for the rally and preparations begin. I continue in my role as adviser. My letter to the editor appears in the *Courant.* They highlight it with a big graphic of an ambulance.

I am getting pulled in a little more than I want to, but I feel I am safe as long as I keep saying I am not going to organize this. I am not an organizer. I want to stay in the background.

Cressy and I talk daily. He keeps the fire stirred up. When the guy who we thought was going to be running the rally has to drop out because his bosses have told him not to get involved, I tell Cressy, "I will not run this thing."

"They're looking to you," Cressy says. "You're the leader, you're the man."

"No, I'm not," I say.

I'm counting on other people and groups to carry the ball, but many who were originally behind the rally get cold feet and drop out. Most decide a quieter approach will work better and cause fewer problems. People are worried about antagonizing the commissioner. It seems everyone is afraid the commissioner will retaliate against them. Because he regulates hospitals, ambulance companies, doctors, nurses, and paramedics, he has enormous power over them, and that power causes fear. Even I fear that he will come after me and find some reason to take my certification away. When the North Central EMS Region backs out, I say that's it. I'm not doing it alone. The rally is off. I'm not going to be the only one up there.

I tell people, "I wasn't going to stand up there by myself. Screw that. Screw that."

I feel enormous relief, but I admit to being a little depressed. A little beaten. It's not like I put myself on the line and then backed off. I got close to the line, then shied away. I spoke up, but I couldn't move the people to action. Just as well.

An emergency physician from Milford, Jay Walshon, calls me and says he's heard about my rally and wants to participate. I tell him the rally's off, I can't get any support. Everyone is heading for the weeds. He urges me to reconsider. Strongly urges. He is practically yelling at me. He sounds personally angry with me for quitting.

Each day I go to work. I do cardiac arrests, room-one traumas, intercepts with volunteer ambulances. In between heart attacks, MVAs, and drunks, I do my part to get people to call the governor's office. They don't know anything about the politics,

most don't even know what a Regional EMS Council is, or
what the state director does. Will this affect my pay? they ask. I
try to explain. I try to tell them the big picture: it is about
building a system that works for the patients. They nod and say
okay, and I dial the number for them, and they leave their mes-
sages. They do it for me, but I sense many are skeptical. The
nature of our work makes EMTs distrustful of authority, of
management, of politics, of people who claim to have control.

I think about my patients—the man having chest pain, the
woman badly injured in a car accident, the child who eats
poison. I help them with my hands. I am there with them. But
what about the larger structure that put me there to help them?
What about the framework that provides the training, takes the
911 call, sends the ambulance, and ensures that I have the right
equipment, that there is a system in place from 911 call to
trauma surgeon, that there is a system to make sense out of
chaos? The system is vital. If a paramedic cares about a single
patient, he has to care about the system, too. The patient is
what we are all about.

Hell, I think. I don't need an army out there, all I need is myself
and a TV camera. So what if the commissioner comes after me,
and I suddenly find myself being investigated? This is America, the land of the free and home of the brave. I am a citizen
and I am unafraid. If I hold the rally, they will come, and if they
don't, at least I won't have this emptiness in my gut, this cer-
tainty that I didn't dare stand up for what I thought was right.

That night I send a message out on the Internet to a group of
a hundred or so EMS people who have been debating what to
do about the cuts at the state office. The rally is on, the capitol
booked, the microphone secured.

I send Betty Morris an e-mail telling her I am going ahead
with the rally because I think it is the right thing to do. A day
later the North Central Region is back on board. "We have always put the patient first," she says, "and if we are out of step
with the other regions, it won't be the first time."

I talk to groups and sign them up. The Connecticut College of Emergency Physicians, the Connecticut College of

Surgeons—Committee on Trauma, the Connecticut Fire Chiefs, the Emergency Nurses Association, the Connecticut Society of EMS Instructors, the Connecticut Sponsor Hospital Clinical Care Coordinators Committee, and many groups and individuals from across the state, including numerous volunteer ambulance services. We are now the Coalition to Save the Connecticut EMS systems. I make up some letterhead on my computer. We are in business.

I write letters to the governor requesting meetings, press advisories go out. Paul Smith, who was the Head of Education at OEMS, and had his position of more than twenty years eliminated the year before, works with me, working the phones, spreading the word.

"You have to come to the rally," I say to Arthur.
"I'll go if we're back from camp in time."

In my dreams, I see a Woodstock of EMS, where I'll stand like Martin Luther King at the Washington Mall, looking out over Bushnell Park, a sea of people in uniforms, backed by ambulances, the Life Star helicopter circling above. I am at the microphone. "I have a dream that one day we will all stand together. Commercial, volunteer, fire, doctor, nurse, EMT, and policeman. We are the colors of the rainbow, red, green, blue, yellow, black and white, we're all equal in God's sight. Common ground! Keep hope alive! Keep hope alive!"

In my nightmares, it is raining, they take our microphone away, and there are only three people there anyway, all of them laughing at this joke of a rally. The commissioner stands there, cackling to himself, then says to me, "Come on, just give me your cert now, let's get it over with, save us both the trouble. What are you worried about? The welfare office is just down the street. Ha ha ha."

Monday arrives. The weather is overcast with periods of showers, but it clears by noon. Slowly, ambulances arrive and a crowd gathers. Maybe sixty to eighty people, most of whom I know. There are a number of local volunteer ambulances. Joe

Schwartz, the director of operations at our company, brings down several ambulances, unexpected support for which I am grateful. The TV stations are here. At high noon, I give the signal for the ambulances to let their sirens run for a minute—a sound bite for the news. I act as MC, giving a brief opening statement, then introducing the speakers—physicians, nurses, fire chiefs. They are very eloquent. They are men and women whom I have worked with at the health department, sat with in countless meetings, witnessed their time volunteered to improve the system.

"I am here as medical control for thirty ambulance services," declares Dr. Ian Cummings of the Eastern Region. "More than that I am here as a citizen, a person whose family is being cared for by the EMS system, a system I am responsible for, a system being decapitated, that is now at threat. Therefore, the people I care about are at threat."

Dr. Mark Quigley of the North Central Region—who, months later, will tragically lose his life after being hit by a car while assisting the victim of a car accident on a dark country road—declares, "The collapse of this system will be a catastrophe for the citizens of Connecticut. The commissioner should be leading us into the next century of EMS, not dragging us toward the last one."

Marty Stillman of the Connecticut Society of EMS Instructors gives a fiery performance. "We're here because we're concerned about patient care. We want to see the best possible patient care. . . . Three million citizens rely on a system when it's a question of life and death. . . . It is a system. It's not just the ambulance that responds or the doctor in the emergency room or the nurse in the emergency room. It's all of us working together to make sure that the emergency medical system provides the best possible patient care. It's all we care about. . . . It's been underfunded, and the people making these decisions don't even know what EMS is about. It's not an economic issue. For the money this state spends on EMS they get a hell of a bargain. A real bargain. But they don't know they're getting a bargain because we haven't told them. We've been too busy providing the best patient care, the best emergency care in the field and in the emergency room. We must educate the public."

The gathering is over in forty-five minutes. Afterward, Dr. Walshon and I go up to see if the governor is in. I have written and called repeatedly but received no answer to my request for a meeting. We stand in the outer office while the secretary eats an apple and talks to someone on the phone. A staffer walks through the gate like I used to when I worked there.

"Is the governor in?" I ask.

"He is in a meeting," the secretary says.

"We'd like to meet with him."

"You can make a request in writing."

"We have," I say.

"Well, let me take your number then."

I give it to her, and we walk back down the stairs. The steps are vacant now. Dr. Walshon and I shake hands. He walks off. I gather my box of press kits and head to my car.

That night the rally is the lead story of the news on Channel 30. Jerry Brooks, the coanchor, begins, "Our top story tonight, a warning from the people who work in the state's emergency medical services program." His coanchor Joanne Nestie continues, "They say if budget cuts go through, their system will collapse and lives will be jeopardized." They cut live to the state capitol where correspondent Tom Monohan says, "EMS workers staged a protest rally outside the state capitol today. They said if there are budget cuts they will not be able to do the best possible job they can. They also said at the current spending levels they have been able to save lives."

The TV then shows two examples of EMS dispatchers helping people save lives.

The correspondent continues. "At the capitol today, doctors, EMS workers and volunteers slammed the proposed cuts." The camera pans the rally, and because it is on the broad back steps, it looks sparsely attended.

They interview Dr. Martin Gross, a surgeon from Stamford hospital, who says, "With the budget cuts that they're going to pull, it will essentially eliminate the ability of the regional councils to function."

They cut back to the correspondent who is shown walking in the health department with the bureau chief of regulation. "But the state says no lives will be jeopardized by any of the cutbacks." They interview the bureau chief who says very matter-of-factly, "When you call nine-one-one, you will continue to access the same quality emergency medical services you currently receive."

And that's it, end of story. It is over and forgotten minutes later as other stories come on: an earthquake in some foreign country, the weather, sports, consumer tips, a health update.

I sit alone. I have a beer, take a bath, get a headache, go to sleep. Exhausted.


The next morning there is an article on page A6 of the *Courant*. The headline reads AT CAPITOL, 60 PROTEST CUTS IN EMERGENCY SERVICES." Sixty, I think. There were at least eighty there, maybe ninety. A hundred.

"How'd the rally go?" Arthur asks.

"It was all right," I say. "There's an article in the paper."

"You're kidding, I missed it." He reads it. "We stayed an extra day at the campground," he says. "Other than a morning shower, it was a beautiful day."

Our first call is for a woman having a seizure. She has fallen and hit her head, so we have to C-spine her. She has never had a seizure before, so we are concerned. At the hospital, while waiting in triage, she says she thinks she's going to throw up. "Art," I yell. He comes down the hall. "Quick," I say. I am at the head. We snap the strap buckles off, and start to turn her so she won't choke on her vomit. I see her cheeks swell and, like a volcano, she projectile vomits straight up. My face is hit with a blast of warm water and vomit.

"I'm sorry," she says.

It covers my glasses and drips from my mustache. I wipe it off with my sleeve and say, that's okay. I give my report to the nurse, and we transfer her over. In the bathroom, I wash my face and mustache.

"The poor paramedic," I hear the woman tell the nurse. "I can't believe I threw up in his face."

We have to go back to the base, where I have a clean shirt in my car.

"I bet that never happened to you when you worked for the state," Arthur says.

"Detail completed," I tell the dispatcher, and we're back on line.

# Shaman

Debbie sees me in the hallway and asks if I am going to the EMS conference sponsored by the Journal of Emergency Medical Services that is coming to Hartford. She says the speakers they have are really good, and it might do me some good to expose myself to them. It is a chance to hear national speakers and to show that Hartford is a town that supports EMS education. It costs $120 for a one-day session, which is all I can do because I play in a softball league on Sundays. I can get education credits for free by attending the regular sessions at Saint Francis, but I think I really should support this, so I go ahead and sign up for the Saturday session.

The conference is excellent, just what I need. I attend three classes, all given by dynamic speakers—it is the Harvard of EMS. One session in particular excites me. It is called "The Path to Professionalism" taught by Scott Bourn, an EMT-Paramedic and longtime educator. He poses the question "What is a paramedic?" and talks about how one day on an airplane he was sitting next to a paramedic. Keeping his own occupation to himself, he asked the paramedic what he did, and the answer was, I do IVs, intubations, needle crics, shock people, and give drugs. He says he has had similar conversations with other medics, and that he finds too many people focus on the tasks and not on the roles. He defines the roles of the paramedic as clinician, caregiver, researcher, influencer, teacher, learner, human, and for each, defines what they mean. I take notes furiously. The kind of paramedic he is talking about is the kind of paramedic I want to be. Sure, I want to get the tubes and do needle crics and chest decompressions, but what he is talking about sounds so much more appealing, so much greater. He talks about how in Florida, the EMS community cut the rate of pediatric drownings in half by studying how they occurred—in many cases the parent went inside for just a moment to answer the telephone. By working with the phone company on a plan to get everyone who has a pool a cellular phone, they cut the rate in half in one year. Think of all those kids, alive today, who will go on and have families of their own, and be doctors, teachers, policeman, paramedics, and live and love and play, rather than have their lives ended as they are pulled blue from the pool and a desperate paramedic struggles to breathe life back into them and wakes at night with the nightmares of their dead faces. *They cut the rate in half.* Imagine being able to say you did something like that. He talks about appreciating the greatness of what we are allowed to do in our job, how daily parents hand us—strangers—their children, what a gift that is, what trust they place in us. How we should be a model by example: walk the walk, take responsibility, initiate change, don't neglect people in your own life, and know what you look like when you stop caring.

In the question-and-answer session, Marge Leticia, the EMS coordinator at New Britain General Hospital, makes a point about healers and shamans of ancient cultures; in a way that is what, at our best, we are. What a privilege to be able to lay our hands on others and try to make them whole.

Some of the stuff may sound sappy, but it inspires me. It makes me want to be a clinician, a caregiver, a researcher, an influencer, a teacher, a learner, a human. And yes, a shaman. (Though I don't think the company would let me wear one of those big masks and carry a long bone stick.) I know it will take more than just the talk to get me back, but it is a lift, a small step. It gives me hope.

# Payback

I come to work, and there in operations are several students in their white shirts, waiting to hook up with paramedics for the day. When I was in paramedic school I rode with paramedics all over the state. Some were great; others were largely silent, acting as if I was an intrusion into their lives and routine. I thought, How could you not treat a rider well? You have limited time to ride, and it is your introduction to the life. Now that I have been a paramedic for several years, I know how they felt. I remember every medic I rode with, but a student who rode with me last month I might not recognize. Sometimes, you just want to go to work, do your job, and not have to put up with anything. Still, I make the effort, because I haven't forgotten my own experience.

Today we get a young girl from Massachusetts named Andrea, who it turns out is from the same program where I took my basic EMT eight years ago, and she knows my old teacher, Judy Moore, who so influenced me. Arthur and I make her feel very welcome. She needs to get a field tube. I haven't had one for a while myself, and I am reluctant to let her do it, if we get one—but I tell her if we do, depending on the patient, I may let her do it.

"I don't want to jeopardize anyone," she says.

"Don't worry," I say.

We're just leaving Windsor when the call comes in for a cardiac arrest at a nursing home right off the highway. We're not two minutes away.

"Let's save a life," I say.

We wheel down the hallway into a room where the staff is doing compressions and bagging the patient. "Go to the head and bag," I say to Andrea. "I'll pass you the stuff in a moment." I put the woman on the monitor. She's in PEA—a rhythm without pulses. I open up the airway kit, and hand Andrea the laryngoscope and the tube with the stylet in it. "Go for it," I say.

I strap a tourniquet around the woman's arm and sink an eighteen-gauge in the antecubital (AC) vein. Arthur hands me the line. Andrea is having a little trouble seeing. "You got it?" I ask. I am tempted to take over, but she sticks with it. "There's peanut butter or something in there," she says. I push my hand on the woman's neck to help drop the cords into view. Andrea has a determined look. She sticks with it and passes the tube. I can feel it under my fingers through the thin cartilage. She inflates the balloon and attaches the bag. We check lung sounds. Solid. "Good job," I say. She beams.

I start firing epi into the IV line, while Andrea bags and Arthur gets the stretcher ready for transport. Suddenly the woman's eyes bolt open, causing us to jump back. We feel for pulses. "We have pulses," the nurse says. We all look around, smiling. Andrea is bagging. Art gives her the thumbs-up. I look at the woman's eyes, shine a light into them. Fixed and dilated.

We wheel her down the hall, get her in the ambulance, and take her to Hartford. She's got a pulse and a blood pressure but is not breathing on her own. No one is home upstairs. They put her on a ventilator. When I turn the paperwork in, I see her husband sitting in the room with her, holding her hand. The doctor has just told him they will have to wait and see, but I know she's not coming back. She was out too long. I find Andrea out in the parking lot. "Great job," I say. "You tubed her like a pro. And a save for your first code. You should be very proud."

She smiles. I remember how good I felt after my first tube. You can't let the patient's ultimate outcome bother you too much. You did your job. She's on her way to helping the world.

Though I didn't get the tube, I helped somebody take a step forward. I grew beyond myself. I have started to repay those who helped me. I feel good.

I look around at the other medics I know, some I am in awe of, some great generous teachers; others are burnt, with broken greatness, what they had once to give now gone. I wonder what will happen to me? Will I be a good teacher? Will I be someone to look up to? A holy shaman? Will I soar above the city or will I crash in flames?

# Rebecca

The company has a new batch of just-certified paramedics who need to be trained. Daniel Tauber, the chief paramedic, and Debbie Haliscak, the EMS coordinator, ask me to precept Rebecca Drotch. I like Rebecca and eagerly agree.

"This will be good for you," Debbie says.

I think it is just what I need. Maybe it will recharge me. Give me perspective. New life. A return to the basics. Break me out of my funk.

Daniel Tauber tells me, "Rebecca's going to need someone with maturity, someone who will instill some discipline in her." They have changed the rules of field training since I was precepted. Now the preceptee must ride as a third so the preceptor can sit with them in the back on the calls, rather than driving and coaching through the rearview mirror. He says Arthur and I are the right people.

Rebecca, while much younger than I was when I precepted, has some advantages I didn't. For the last year she has worked regularly with paramedics. Some have even let her run calls under their watchful eyes. I have worked with her myself several times. Her IV skills are excellent, and her assessments are strong. We have a good time together and joke easily with each other.

* * *

Rebecca will be the first person I have precepted, and I have to admit the night before I feel a bit of nervousness. What if we get the really bad call? How can I teach her if I myself am being taxed? I don't know everything, and I think maybe that will be my approach—what I know I can teach her, what I don't we can learn together. The morning we start I tell her what my preceptor, Tom Harper, told me, that whatever happens is between us, and I will never say anything bad about her to anyone.

"Thanks," she says. "I know you wouldn't."

The truth is she has little of the fear about failing that I did. She's worked around medics enough to see the good ones and the mediocre ones, and she knows she will be at least as good as some.

"How long do you think it will take?" she asks. "I'd like to get done in six weeks. Four would be better. It can't go over eight. That would be awful."

I tell her it all depends on what kind of calls we get. We need to do a cardiac arrest. Other than that, all I am really looking for is to see that she is comfortable and that her thought pattern is working the right way. I will not be a drill sergeant. I hear of another preceptor who tells his preceptee, "Two rules: first, the preceptor is always right; two, see rule number one." I do not want Rebecca to be a robot of my own making. I want her to find her own style; I want her to have confidence. After she has finished her first checklist, I say, "Let's go out and do some good."

Our first call is for an unresponsive man at a nursing home in East Hartford. We find him sitting at the nursing station, being held in the chair by a nurse. His eyes look glazed. His forehead is cool and clammy. Rebecca asks the nurse what he is like normally. She replies that he's normally alert and oriented. Rebecca looks at me for a moment. I give her a you're-the-boss-don't-look-at-me look. "Why don't we get him going?" she says.

"Sounds good."

We put him on the stretcher, and put on an oxygen mask. In

the elevator, she feels his pulse. "He's bradycardic." In the ambulance, she gets a pressure of 60. He is in a junctional rhythm
of 40 on the monitor. His pulse saturation is in the 60s, but it
could be because his pressure is so low, he's not perfusing to
his extremities so we are getting a bad read. "What do you
want to do?" I ask.

"Start a line."

"Good idea. Why don't you look on that arm and I'll look on
this one?" I find a vein that looks good and say, "I got one."

"I got one, too," she says. "Give me an eighteen."

She makes it clear that she is going to do the IV, so I stand
back. Nothing wrong with aggressiveness. I keep my eye on
the vein I found in case she misses, but she gets it right away
and draws up the blood. I hand her the line, and she says,
"Open wide?"

"Yup. What else do you want to do?"

"Give him a bolus?"

"How about something for his rate?"

"Atropine?"

"Good choice."

I open the drug box, hand her a bristojet and a vial of atropine. The bristojet is a special syringe the vial screws into.
She looks at me, and holding one in each hand, flips the yellow
tops off with her thumbs, like they used to do on the old TV
show *Emergency*, which I saw when it was first on and she has
only seen in reruns. She smiles. "I had to do it," she says.

"High marks on your technique," I say. It is a rite of passage
for all paramedics, flipping the tops and sending them spinning
through the air.

She pushes the atropine. "Fast," I tell her.

We are crossing the river now, headed to Saint Francis on a
priority two. The man's rate jumps up to 112. She checks a
pressure and hears it well at 130/70.

We both look at the patient. He is still unresponsive. His
blood sugar checked out fine. His respiratory rate is about ten
and shallow. I look out the window. We're about six blocks
from the hospital. I am thinking I wish we were ten blocks

away. I look at Rebecca. "Do you know what I'm thinking?" I see a gleam in her eye.

"Tube him?" she says.

"Go for it."

I almost tell Arthur to swing around the block a couple times. She opens the airway kit, while I get the ambu-bag out for her. She goes in with the laryngoscope, and I press down against his Adam's apple to try to bring the cords down into view. "Only do it if you see them," I say.

I am thinking, she's not going to get it, but at least I'm letting her try.

"If you don't see them, pull out, and we need to bag him."

"I got 'em," she says. She has a look of fierce determination on her face, as if she's about to get into a fistfight. She goes in with the tube. I can feel it pass beneath the skin under my fingers. "I'm in," she says. She pulls out the stylet.

We are in the driveway of the hospital now. She tapes the tube down, and we check for placement by listening to lung sounds. "You're in," I say. "Congratulations."

She beams.

"First call, you get a tube," I say. "Too much."

When we pull him out on the stretcher, other medics and EMTs who have been standing there all stop talking to watch us. Everyone watches a new preceptee, everyone wants to know how she's doing. Here's Rebecca on her first call, bagging the tubed patient. She is smiling, her face flushed as if she was just named woman of the year. Afterward people will come up to me, ask if she was the one who got the tube, and I'll say yes, she did. I brag about her for the rest of the day. I didn't get the IV or the tube, but I helped her. It may take getting used to, but it feels good.

The first week goes well. Rebecca is comfortable in the job, and has a good knowledge base. She needs little help from me, doing all nine IVs by herself without a miss. I get after her to be more thorough with her morning checklist and try to teach her there is a higher standard of conduct now that she is a paramedic. We bring in a fifty-three-year-old man with chest pain radiating down his left arm since last night. His vital signs are okay, but he appears scared, and when we put him on the monitor, he has ST elevation, which is a good indicator he is having a heart attack. Rebecca gets the line, puts him on oxygen, gives him some baby aspirin and a nitro.

When we wheel him into triage, the triage nurse is taking a report from another paramedic. An ER tech sees Rebecca and gives her a hug, then says he has to tell her something and pulls her into the EMT room just a few feet from the triage area. I look at the patient and see the fear in his eyes. What she has done—forgetting about her patient's emotional need—is something I have also done in the past, but now standing against the wall I recognize this failure. When Rebecca comes back a moment later, I glare at her, but she doesn't notice.

Afterward I scold her. "I'm upset with you," I say.

"What'd I do? I didn't do anything wrong. I didn't miss anything, did I? What? Tell me."

"You abandoned your patient. This guy was having an MI. He was scared and frightened, you were joking around with the tech, and you abandoned him." She looks a little stunned. Everything has been going so well, and now the first criticism.

"I didn't mean to, but he pulled me away."

"It was unprofessional. You've got to just say no. You're a paramedic now. Take care of your patient."

"But I didn't mean to."

"No buts. Don't do it again."

She frowns, wounded.

I feel like a preceptor now. I have found fault, but I can't keep up the heavy role. "Look, you're doing great, just remember not to do it the next time. You always need to be aware of your patient."

We get sent for chest pain to the state capitol, where a protestor has experienced some chest tightness in the heat of a rally. I always feel a little uneasy going into the capitol on a call, because there is a crowd of people watching you, and I wonder how many recognize me from when I used to work for the former governor and wonder what I am doing. We take in all the equipment and are led to a room off the main corridor, where the man sits in a chair. He looks a little ashen, but says he is all right, his heart is just beating a little fast—he has a problem with that. His pulse is too fast to count. We put him on the monitor and he is going at 240.

"What do you want to do?" I ask Rebecca.

"Adenosine," she says, lighting up.

"You want me to do the line for you?"

"No, I'll do it," she says, and pushes right by me.

With adenosine, you need to get a good-sized vein as high up as possible because of the short half-life of the drug. She gets the line and tells the patient he may feel something unpleasant. He says he's had it before, but it hasn't worked. He says the first time the paramedics had to shock him. I am thinking, as much as I want Rebecca to get her skills, I hope not. I have seen conscious people shocked; it is not pleasant to watch.

The first six doesn't touch him.

I draw up twelve and hand it to Rebecca. This time it does the trick, and his rate converts to 112.

"You saved my life," he says, looking at Rebecca as if he is in love with her. "You're the best."

She is smiling; Arthur and I are standing around like big lugs.

We get the stretcher ready, and I pick up the trash, the IV wrappers and empty drug vials and needles.

Suddenly the man says, "I'm not feeling so well." His head drops face forward onto the desk. We both look at the monitor. He is ventricular tachycardia—a lethal rhythm. I reach for the fast patch pads and am considering just punching him in the chest to set the heart back to a sustainable rhythm. I am cursing that we don't have him on the stretcher. He's a big guy; it's going to be hard to manhandle him from behind the desk.

He lifts his head up. "Wow," he says.

I look back at the monitor. He has broken back on his own.

"You all right?"

"Yeah, I just went out."

I look at Arthur, and we both raise our eyebrows.

"There you are, little pretty," he says to Rebecca. "My

savior. What's your name? I'm going to write a letter to your boss."

He is stable all the way to the hospital.


We are together a month, and after a while, it is like I am not there. She is competent, she gets all her IVs, and the job is becoming routine. What we are waiting for is a cardiac arrest, a requirement to complete precepting. I try to trip her up, by taking stuff out of the equipment, and seeing if she finds it. After nailing her a few times—no ambu-bag, no BP cuff—she gets on to me. Then one day I put a note in the spare equipment box, which says *Hey, Rebecca! How's the checklist going?* I ask her if she checked the spare box, and she says she did. I ask her what she found and she hems and haws. "You didn't check it," I say.

"I did, but—"

"You didn't check it."

"I did. I did. I didn't find anything. What did I miss?"

At the end of the day I give her her first bad evaluation. *Rebecca continues to do well with her assessment, skills, etc. The lack of challenging calls is hindering the conclusion of her precepting, and it raises the question of her ability to maintain focus. The improvements she needs most to make are within herself in terms of day-to-day commitment to all the standards of a professional, mature paramedic and person.*

After she reads it, she gives me a half-glare, half–hurt look and then punches out. When I say, "We'll get them next week," she says nothing but keeps going out the door.


The next week, we climb into the back of a volunteer service ambulance just off the highway. The man on the stretcher has a huge stomach and is breathing at a rate of six a minute. Unresponsive. Fifty years old, found on the couch by his daughter, a history of heavy drinking. The volunteers called for a medic as soon as they arrived, loaded him, and hit the road for the intercept point. They are bagging him, breathing for him by squeezing a plastic bag attached to the oxygen supply. Still, he is blue from the neck up—he needs an airway. Rebecca goes to the head to intubate, while I put him on the monitor. After looking all over for a vein, I feel one in his hand and hit it on my first try. Rebecca's having trouble with the tube. The man has a squat neck, and his mouth is filled with bloody secretions. She tries to pass it, but it goes in the stomach, not the trachea. We have to pull it. She goes in again with the laryngoscope, struggling to lift up the tongue and sweep it to the side so she can get a view of the cords. She suctions to see. A wave of fetid blood comes out, and I can see her fighting back the urge to vomit. She wants the tube so bad, but she can't get it.

"We need to bag him," I say.

She pulls out and we ventilate.

I give him some dextrose, while Rebecca draws up some Narcan, which we also push through the IV, but neither works.

I notice the man's stomach seems to have gotten bigger. It was large and distended when we got in.

"It's been getting bigger since we found him," one of the volunteers says.

"Let's get out of here now," I say. I don't know if it's the air from bagging him or if he has some major abdominal bleed, which is probably more likely given the dark blood in his mouth. And if it is a bleed, we've wasted valuable time at the intercept point. He needs a surgeon.

As we bounce and hurtle toward the hospital, Rebecca tries again for the tube, but she can't get it. I switch places and try myself, but we are almost there, and I can't see a thing amid the dark blood and vomit in his mouth. We suction and keep bagging. His stomach keeps swelling.

At the hospital, he isn't in the cardiac room five minutes before his heart rate plunges and he codes—flatline. They fire epi and atropine into the IV line, while a nurse does compressions on his chest. They call an anesthesiologist to come down and intubate him. The anesthesiologist looks at the patient and shakes his head. He suctions the airway, then passes the tube on his first attempt, but by now it is too late. They work him another ten minutes, but he is gone.

Later, after I have washed my hands, I walk by the cardiac room and see Rebecca in there alone, standing over the gurney looking down at the man's body. Standing next to her now, I know what she is thinking. I have thought it myself many times. I failed you. Your life was in my hands. I let you down. You died because of my failure. Her eyes are wet. I know just what she is thinking. What she is feeling.

I put my hand on her shoulder. "Come on," I say.

We walk down the hall silently. It is a walk that we take many times a day without even noticing it, but this time the hall seems longer, darker, like a runway out of the stadium after a big game we have lost. You feel great, you feel confident, then *wham*, you get knocked down so low you can't stand it. Darkness closes in on you. Doubt is all-consuming. Others start to say "hi," but they can see it in our faces now, and they know not to talk.

We reach the automatic doors, go outside, and sit down on the curb.

"I thought I was ready," she says. "It was all coming so easy. This sort of set me back, shook me to reality. He needed a tube, and I couldn't get it. There was nothing more we could do. It was horrible knowing there was nothing. Unless I could have gotten the tube."

I have taught her several things in our time together—to be thorough, to do your assessment, to take nothing for granted, to be in tune with your patient's emotional as well as their medical needs, to let your patients talk and to listen, but this is the most difficult lesson.

"Let me tell you a secret," I say. "You're never going to be ready. You're going to have calls that kick your butt, and this one kicked ours. It's what being a paramedic is about. You learn no matter how good you are, it's often not going to be enough."

"If only I'd gotten the tube."

"We didn't get it. You don't always get it. And it feels bad. It should feel bad. You understand what I saying?"

"Not really."

"What we do matters, so when we fail it hurts. The bad calls never go away—they live with you. That guy is going to make you better, and he'll be with you, they'll all be with you, helping you when you're performing miracles, when you're saving people you have no right to save."

"Yeah?"

"Yeah, and you didn't kill this guy—he was on his way out before we even got there. You are going to save lives. You'll save them because you are a paramedic and a decent one. Trust me on that."

She looks up at me as I stand. She blinks, wondering maybe if what I say is true, wanting to believe.

"Now, finish up your paperwork. We have some good to do yet today."

"Okay," she says. "Thanks."

"You did all right," I say.

As I walk away, I think, she's just like me.

We get our code at a nursing home in Bloomfield—a ninety-four-year-old man last seen awake an hour before. CPR is in progress when we arrive. Everything goes like clockwork. Rebecca gets the tube, I get the line. She runs through the algorithm, epi and atropine. We get a rhythm back on the way to the hospital, but no pulses. Outside the hospital, I let Rebecca do an EJ—an external jugular vein IV—which she does perfectly.

I recommend that she be able to ride alone with me now. Arthur gets shipped out to work a BLS transfer car. Rebecca does great. We intercept with a crew for an unresponsive male, and it's like I'm not even there. Rebecca assesses the patient, gets the line, checks the blood sugar, and fires in some dextrose, and the man is awake and talking.

My job is to drive, remake the stretcher after every call, clean and restock the ambulance. I never realized just how much physical labor is involved in being a paramedic's partner. We go into a call and assess the patient, then she tells me to get the stair chair. I have to lug the stretcher out by myself, set it up, get out the stair chair, carry it upstairs, help her carry the patient down, gather the rest of the equipment, and then while she works on the patient, put the stair chair back in. One habit she hasn't improved is she makes a mess in the back. IV wrappers and four-by-fours all over the place. Blood on the floor, which I have to spray down and wipe clean with serious elbow grease.

I see Arthur bringing in a transfer. "How's it going?" he asks.

"She's working me like a dog," I say. "Like an animal."

"Now you know how the rest of us live," he says.

It's 6:50 and Rebecca wants to head in so she can prepare for her date that night. "We've got another call left," I say. "Shooting on Albany Avenue, another ten minutes."

"Yeah, right," she says.

At 6:55, the HPD radio crackles. "Four-seven-one."

"Four-seven-one."

"Four-seven-one, on a one, Homestead Avenue for the shooting."

"You were right," she says.

"Off by a street."

We arrive to a chaotic scene. Hundreds of people have gathered. To the left I can see a body on the ground by the hedges. Yet several people shout, "This way, in the house."

"No, over here, over here," a woman shouts, pointing to the guy on the ground.

"Check him out," I say to Rebecca.

I get on the radio. "We need another ambulance. We've got one victim on the street, and they say there's another in the house."

Rebecca is kneeling by the man, who lies facedown on the pavement. His baggy pants have fallen down around his knees, his butt is bare to the sky.

"He's dead," she says.

I've brought the stretcher and long board, and we roll him onto the board. A woman is screaming, "Is he all right? Is he all right?"

His face is bloody, but I can't see a bullet hole, though one nostril looks a little bigger than the other. He is not breathing and has no pulse. We get him on the board and lift him onto the stretcher.

"Come with me," another woman shouts, pulling at my sleeve. "He's in the house. He's bleeding."

"There's another ambulance coming," I say.

We wheel him low and fast back to the ambulance. "You tube him, I'll get the line," I say to Rebecca.

We get him in the back, and while Rebecca goes for the tube, I cut off his clothes, looking for bullet holes, but find none. I stick a fourteen in his left AC, press against his Adam's apple as Rebecca passes the tube. On the monitor he is in an agonal rhythm. On the radio I hear them scrambling to get a third ambulance. "We need help," Rebecca says. "Anyone."

"You're doing this by yourself," I say. I open up the biotech and pull out the epi. "We're just a couple minutes from Saint Fran. Bag, drug, CPR. You can do it."

I jump out and get in the driver's seat. The ambulance has been taped in by police tape. I swing around and yell at a cop to move his car so I can get through. I break through the police tape and head out lights and sirens. I pass the second, then the third ambulance. I patch to Saint Fran. "Approximately twenty-year-old male, gunshot to the head, in traumatic arrest, patient intubated, line in place, CPR in progress. Out in one minute."

They have help out front for us. I open the door to see the police tape is hanging off the ambulance in streamers; it looks like a limo carrying newlyweds. We get the patient into the trauma room where the full team is waiting. They inspect him, while taking over CPR. "How do you know he's shot?" a surgeon asks.

I really don't know what to say to that. We got sent for a shooting, there were a hundred people there, shouting about people shot. This is a twenty-year-old male, otherwise healthy, lying facedown on the ground, with a mask on, his butt naked to the sky, not breathing, no pulse. No wounds other than blood on his face. I don't think he died of old age. "One nostril looks a little bigger than the other," I say. "There could be two more victims coming in."

I shake Rebecca's hand. "Good job."

"I can't believe I did it myself."

"We couldn't wait around."

Fifteen minutes later, the other ambulance comes in with the other victim—there is only one other—who has a bad leg wound with arterial bleeding and no blood pressure. They have four people in the back with them. He codes in the trauma room, but they get him back.

The families converge on the hospital, holding each other, wailing. I tell Rebecca, "Look at them. Sometimes you think these people are scumbags, but they all have families and are loved."

"I know, I almost cried when we got there. That was his mother standing over him."

I didn't even notice that. All I was thinking was here is this young gangbanger who died bare butt to the sky, baggy pants around his knees—a drawback of the latest fashion. I didn't even think that the woman was anybody but a person getting in my way. Rebecca knew it was his mother. I look at her and she has tears in her eyes. I look back at the family and am ashamed that I feel nothing. Here I am trying to teach a lesson of compassion, which is hollow because my own is gone. I look at Rebecca and see what I have forgotten.

In our final days together while we wait for Rebecca to ride with Debbie or Daniel to get final clearance, I try to get back to what a paramedic is really about. She has all the skills and medicine down. We help a cancer patient's family work through an insurance problem so the patient can get transported to the right hospital. Even though it takes almost an hour on scene, we get the problem solved. We help an old woman who has fallen and can't get up by herself get back into bed, then get her some food and rearrange her furniture to make her life a little easier. Another woman fell in the bathroom and defecated on herself. We clean her up and get her in fresh clothes, rather than dumping her on the stretcher in what she was wearing.

I go in on a Friday to pick up my paycheck and see Daniel Tauber, who mentions that he will be riding with Rebecca on

Tuesday to give her clearance. I almost call Rebecca to give her a heads up, but then think she'll enjoy the weekend more without worrying about how she'll do. I am confident she'll do fine.

On Tuesday, I am back with Art. "She wore me out."

"I'm glad you know what it's like to be a paramedic's partner," he says.

"Yes, it was good. I learned a few things. You can be quicker if you don't wash your hands. And taking a pee costs you probably ninety seconds, so I'm going to institute new rules for you."

He laughs.

"It's good to be back together," I say. "Not that I didn't enjoy it, but I was getting a little rusty."

"Yes, it is," he says.

We listen over the radio and hear Rebecca and Daniel go out to a difficulty breathing, and later a chest pain. I see her in the afternoon and things are going well. She gets cut loose—a paramedic in her own right.

"I feel like a father," I say to Arthur.

"You did well," he says. "She'll make us proud."


# A Paramedic Again


It's nine o'clock and we've already done two calls when we get sent to back up 866, another medic unit, on a Macing. Five police cars, an ambulance, and a fire truck are on scene. I get out and ask Todd Beaton, the medic, what we can do for him. His eyes are red. I see now that his partner, Shawn Wood, and their paramedic student rider also have red eyes. "You have any more saline?" he asks.

Are you guys the patients?" I ask.

He shakes his head. "No, we're all right. The patient's in the police car. We couldn't get in. The cops broke down the door. The guy looked postictal, like he was coming around from a seizure, and he came at one of the cops, and we all ended up getting Maced."

"You all right?"

"We're better now."

I go over to the police car, where I see a handcuffed bare-chested man with eyes swelled nearly shut and drool all over his face and chest. Two cops are standing by the car. "What do you want us to do with this guy?" I ask.

The female cop says, "I want you to treat him." She opens the door.

"You're going to have to uncuff him," I say.

"No, I'm not, he's under arrest."

"He's not going in my ambulance cuffed unless you're coming with me."

"You can treat him in the police car."

"No, I can't treat him in the police car. He had a seizure. He needs to go to the hospital."

"What if he escapes? Are you willing to be responsible?"

The other cop comes over.

"Look," I say. "These medics, who I trust, say he appeared postictal, indicating he had a seizure. He needs to go to the hospital. I can't take him cuffed, unless one of you is going to ride in the back with me."

"He had a seizure?" the cop says.

"Yes, I believe so."

"Then he's all yours. That's all I want to know." He pulls him out of the car and hands him over to me.

"He needs to be uncuffed."

"She'll get the key."

Todd and Shawn are feeling better now, so I turn over the patient. The cop gets in their ambulance and uncuffs the patient. Once he's on the stretcher, Shawn pours saline in the patient's eyes.

I say to Todd, "And you were complaining about not getting

on line. Welcome back to the city." The company finally responded to our complaints, and while the "dead-icated" system is still in place, they have increased the number of paramedic cars on line, and have reiterated their goal to put a medic in every car as soon as possible. Three new sets of medic gear—monitors, drug boxes, airway kits, appear at operations.

"How do you like it now?" I say to Todd.

He just shakes his head.

I learn later that the patient had wrestled with the cop and was reaching for his gun when Todd grabbed him. Then the cop Maced him, the spray nipping Todd and everyone else in the room.

We're sent for a car accident on West Service Road, which is a circular road off I-91, just north of the city. The dispatcher says he thinks its down by the old Howard Johnson's. We get off Jennings Road and head left to where HoJo's is, but when we get there, we find it's been flattened. Nothing but rubble, a few bright orange tiles visible amid the brick and dirt. It looks like Oklahoma City. "Oh my God," I say, pretending to speak into the mike, "Mayday, Mayday."

"Maybe we should ask if they've had any reports of explosions," Art says.

We can't find a motor vehicle accident anywhere.

"It's by the Oldsmobile place," the dispatcher comes back. "They called it in."

"Oh great, a fender-bender in the parking lot," Art says. We spin around and head to the dealership but can't see anything. A salesman comes out and points down the road. "Down that way," he says. "One of our cars was involved." At the same time, over the radio, the dispatcher says, "We're getting calls from the highway, there's a car on its side just off the road."

We race down the road. Ahead we see a vehicle on its side against the fence, people lying in the road.

"We've got it," Art says. "We've got bodies all over the place."

I get out and quickly note that no one appears badly hurt, but it is a strange sight. People are lying in the road like participants in a casualty drill, all except one man—wearing baggy pants and a snowjacket even though the temperature is in the sixties—who sits against the fence, shouting into his cellular phone. Nearby a brand-new 4-Runner, its windows all smashed out, is on its side against a fence. "Pick me up and get your fuckin' ass out here," the man on the phone says, waving his hands about like a rap singer. There are three other similarly dressed people lying on the ground. Two of them are also on cellular phones.

In the middle of the road is a skinny man in a white shirt and tie, wearing glasses. "I'm a little bit shook up," he says, with a rapid Pakistani accent, "but I think I'm okay. They told me not to move so I been lying here still as I can be."

"Well, what happened?"

"I told dem to slow down, but dey went faster instead. Then de car went ober and ober. I thought it was the end for this berson. Oh, I'm going to lose my job."

I go back to the ambulance to radio that we have four minor injuries and will need a second ambulance. The cavalry is already on the way. Daniel Tauber is coming in a fly car and another ambulance has been coming priority one. Slow it down, I say.

A Bronco pulls up. The man who has been standing against the fence says something to a man on the ground, then gets in the car, which peels out. A police car is coming down the road, followed by a TV news van, an ambulance, and the fly car.

I take two of the younger men in my ambulance, while the other car takes the salesman and the third guy.

"I can't believe this, man," one guy says to the other.

"I ain't going to pay for that, am I?" the driver says, as we head to the hospital. "That ought to be on their license . . . right?"

"They probably have insurance," I say.

"Damn right. That car handles for shit."

We're still laughing about the call when we clear the hospital. On the radio a basic crew is shouting for a medic. They have a cardiac arrest. We are about to volunteer to back them up when the dispatcher Laura Howe calls Rebecca's number—her car is closer.

"Her first code on her own," I say.

"She'll do fine," Arthur says.

Car 875 calls us to assist them at an elderly housing unit. There we find a five-hundred-pound, sixty-year-old female wearing only a cotton robe, sitting on the floor by her bed. She looks like Jabba the Hut's big sister. She had been trying to get off her bed and onto her mobile cart when she fell. She is unable to get up by herself and is too heavy for Faith Creer and Cindy Hudson to lift. Arthur and I each grab her under her shoulders and try to stand her up, but we don't move her an inch. We stop because we are worried we will pull her shoulders out of joint. After numerous attempts, I finally squat down and put my arms around her chest. While our rider grabs her legs and Art a shoulder, I squeeze my arms tight. My arms disappear into her rolls of fat. As I drive my legs up and Art and the rider strain, we move her up against the bed. Art and I go flying on top of her, then she starts to slip back and I catch her with my leg. She slides down on my leg, but I hold it tight to keep her from hitting the floor. She reeks of BO and other smells. My leg feels damp. I can barely see it; folds of fat and both legs hide it. We push up, Art and the rider each holding a leg and my arms in a bear hug around her. We get her completely on the bed. Her house is disgusting and she has no business living there alone, but she doesn't want to leave, and we can't take her against her will. We leave the crew of 875 to get the refusal. We clear, but I ask to return to base to do laundry. I have been pissed on, puked on, bled on, and spit on. I have wiped shit off old ladies' bottoms on numerous occasions, but when I look down at my pant leg now and see it covered with slime and gray pubic hairs and feel its dampness, I am nauseated.

At the base, I put my pants in the washer and pour in two cups full of soap. When I take my pants out, they are foamy white. I wash the soap out in the shower, ring them out, and toss them in the dryer. An hour later, my pants are hot and dry, but I feel only slightly better.

As we walk to the car, Rebecca and her partner pull in. They need to resupply after their code.

"Rebecca, my pride and joy," I say. "How'd it go? Did you get the tube?"

"I got the tube," she says, "and the save."

"All right! A save!"

"I did you proud," she says.

"No doubt."

I want to stay and hear all the details, but we have to get back on the road—the city is hopping with emergencies.

It is one of the busiest days I've worked. We keep banging out the calls. I keep Arthur on the go. I'm whipping out run forms in a matter of minutes, clearing the hospital lickety-split, because they are short of cars. "Let me just go to the bathroom before you clear," Art says.

"But you went this morning," I say.

We do an old woman who fell and broke her wrist. "You're such nice young men," the woman says to Arthur.

"He's not," Arthur tells her. "He is my nemesis. An evil man."

It is the only call I let him tech because he is slow with the paperwork. We are going to Hartford Hospital and I know I will have time to run across the street to the Children's Hospital cafeteria to grab one of the cheap lunch specials, get it eaten, and be back in the rig before he's done, which proves to be the case. "Maybe we'll get a chance to eat before the next call," he says.

"Eat, who needs to eat?" I say. "Suck it in. There are people out there in distress."

He shakes his head and growls. I grab the mike, clear us, and we are immediately sent to Park Street for a maternity. The address is barely three blocks from the hospital. In most maternities we do in the city, the woman meets us at the curb, walks to the ambulance, and hops in back; we drive her to the hospital, we wheel her upstairs, and she gets off, hops onto the table, and delivers within the hour. I make a comment—What, they can't walk two blocks? Art agrees.

The woman is coming down the stairs, wobbling. We get her on the stretcher, and she tells us she is twenty-three weeks pregnant. She was just at the hospital and they sent her home. "The baby is coming," she says. "I got to go to the bathroom. Oh, this pain. Don't let my baby die. All the others, they always die. This always happens. Oh, the pain is killing me. I am Caesarean," she says.

Once we are in the ambulance, I check her to see if the baby is crowning. No sign yet, but the woman is screaming. I tell Arthur, just go. I really want to deliver a baby, but at twenty-three weeks, the baby cannot survive. I remember the one I did deliver, twenty-six weeks, and I never want to go through that again.

"It's coming, it's coming," she says. "I can't take the pain. Don't let this happen."

We're out at Hartford a minute later. We take her right upstairs to labor and delivery, where her screams take a moment to get the staff's attention.

"She was here earlier, twenty-three weeks pregnant. History of three miscarriages. Says she has to go to the bathroom."

Their look that says, What, back again? changes quickly. We wheel her into a delivery room and seven or eight doctors and nurses, quickly gowning up, enter the room. "She's about to deliver," a woman says who has briefly examined her.

"She's going to lose the baby," I say to Arthur.

"What a shame."

I don't even have time to write up the paperwork. They are screaming for cars, so I just clear. They send us out to I-84 East, near the Capitol Avenue exit to assist another car with an MVA. We fight through traffic with Arthur slamming the air horn and traffic turning right in front of us, or stopping dead, and generally causing Arthur to shout and slam the air horn more.

When we arrive on scene, I see that Daniel Tauber, the chief paramedic, and Pat O'Brien, one of the supervisors, are the crew. Daniel comes over; he is really angry. "There is not a scratch on the car," he says, "and this woman wants her and her three kids to be checked out. They all have to be boarded and collared."

On the radio we hear there is a child struck by a car over on

Nelson. No cars are available for several minutes. One finally clears Hartford and must race completely across town to respond, while two units are stuck up here on the highway for bullshit. Daniel takes the mother and the youngest child, while Art and I take the other two girls, ages eleven and five.

At the hospital, I see Daniel has done a mummy job on the woman. He has tape across her eyebrows, three belts on, tape around her velvet dress, tape around her suede shoes. She is incapable of any movement except breathing. She could be turned upside down on the board and not move a inch. One of my little girls has already escaped from my C-spine job, and someone has given her a lollipop. She is sitting on her board, telling her sister that the hospital looks just like it does on TV.

As soon as we clear, we get called for chest pain. I find a fifty-year-old man, alert but lying on the floor. He is pale, ashen, diaphoretic. I give him two baby aspirin to chew. I can't feel a pulse or a BP. His wife and daughter stand in the kitchen doorway, scared. I throw him on a nonrebreather and tell Arthur to get the stretcher. The monitor shows him in a sinus bradycardia at 20. I put in an IV right there, slam in a milligram of atropine. "Are we going to the hospital?" he asks.

"This may help," I say.

The rate comes up to 60. When we get him in the ambulance, I hear a blood pressure of 100. I run the fluid wide open because his lungs are clear. He still has chest pain, but his breathing is a little better. I give him a nitro under the tongue and call the hospital. I tell them what I have and ask for orders for morphine if I can get his blood pressure up with the fluid. They grant it. I give him another nitro and four milligrams of morphine as Arthur races through traffic. I put in another IV line. His pressure is up to 120. He says he's feeling better, though he still has some pain. I give him another nitro. When we hit the ER, they have a room ready with a crew of doctors who descend on him. The ECG confirms the infarct. They put him on heparin, a nitro and morphine drip, and within ten minutes have him upstairs for a catherization to clear out his blocked arteries. I see his wife and child in the waiting room; I bring them in so the doctors can explain what is going on. His wife squeezes my hand and says, "Thank you."

While I am writing up my paperwork, I call dispatch for times. They ask if we can do a call on Willard—there is an unconscious party there and they're out of cars. Willard is just down the street. "Sure," I say.

"Arthur," I shout as I come out of the security room. I see him in the supply closet off the hall. "We've got a call. Did you get a board in?"

"Yes, another call?"

"Hi-ho Silver," I say. We get in the rig. "Unconscious on Willard. They were out of cars."

"Am I surprised?"

A man meets us at the curb.

"What's up?"

"It's my brother. He was on the couch, then all of a sudden, he had trouble breathing."

"How old is he?"

"Thirty-seven."

"What kind of history does he have?" Code for Does he do drugs?

"He's got heart problems."

We get in the elevator. To fit the stretcher in, we have to lift the back to the sitting position. "Is he still breathing?" Arthur asks.

"Yeah, he's breathing."

"Sometimes they don't tell us, so I like to ask."

We get off at the third floor. The door opens and we are face-to-face with a dresser, a few rolled carpets, and a gilded mirror. "Excuse us," I say to the young woman who is obviously moving out. I help her move the mirror and carpets. "Please keep this elevator free for a little. We're going to be needing it."

"Okay," she says, but as soon as we are by, she starts loading the furniture in.

We go down the hall a few doors and follow the man in. We leave the stretcher in the hall. I go in first carrying the monitor. Art has the bag. We go down a narrow hallway and turn into the bedroom. On the far side of the bed, a man lies on a couch. I walk over and look at him.

He is a tall young man. I look at him closely. It is one of those moments that seem to take several minutes, but in reality only lasts a split second, as my eyes tell my mind, my mind thinks on it and processes it, and then I say aloud, "Arthur, he is not breathing."

We pick him up and carry him over to the other side of the bed, where we will set him down on the floor. We need a hard surface to make the CPR compressions effective. "Did he do any heroin today?" I ask.

"No, well, maybe some this morning," his brother says.

We set him down and Art cuts his shirt off, while I put him on the monitor. He is in v-fib. "I have to shock him," I say. I set the dial for 200 joules.

I shock him. His body flinches. I look at the monitor. He is in an idio-ventricular rhythm. I get the airway kit out while Arthur gets on the radio. "Four-seven-one, we have a working one hundred," he says.

Dispatch comes back saying they are sending a crew. I know that means Daniel and Pat because they are just up the street. I stick the stylet into a number-eight tube, attach the ten cc syringe to the end, and then go in for the tube. I see the cords, easily pass the tube.

I listen for breath sounds, equal and positive, negative over the stomach. "I'm in."

I glance at the monitor. He is back in v-fib. I shock him again. This time at 300 joules. His body flinches. Again, we get a rhythm. I feel for pulses. Nothing. Arthur starts compressions again. I recruit the cop who has arrived to handle the ambu-bag. I get some drugs out of my bag, and squirt some epi and atropine down the tube.

We hear the door open, and Daniel and Pat come in with their med kit and a backboard.

"What do we have, gentlemen?" Daniel says.

"Thirty-seven-year-old heroin user. History of heart problems. He was having trouble breathing, his brother says. We found him not breathing. In v-fib, shocked twice. I've just given some epi and atropine down the tube."

"I'll get a line," he says, stepping over me.

We work him hard. I give Narcan in case it was a heroin overdose. More epi, atropine, and lidocaine. Daniel gets two lines going, running full fluid. We shock him nine times, occasionally getting a rhythm, but never a pulse. It is very hot in the apartment and we are all dripping sweat. Finally, he's gone flatline.

"Let's get him out of here," I say. We secure him to the board, tuck his hands in his pants to keep them from flailing. He is a tall man; his feet stick off the end of the board. Arthur and I pick him up, perform several maneuvers to get out of the tight room and finally into the hall, where the stretcher is set up. We resume compressions and bagging in the hall as we roll down to the elevator. The lady moving in has gone with her furniture, but the elevator is not there. We hit the button and wait.

"He's not going to fit in there," Arthur says.

"We can lean the stretcher."

"It's going to be tight."

We push the stretcher in and try to turn it, but the end won't clear the door. I try to lift the back, but it won't give. I have to loosen the straps on the man, then pull hard. We push the stretcher, but the door still won't close. Daniel and I both lift. The stretcher is only on two wheels now, and the man is leaning at a thirty-degree angle. The door starts to close, but it catches his feet. Daniel pulls them in, and I push the elevator door, which scrapes against the foot of the stretcher. Finally, the door closes.

We push the first-floor button, but the elevator goes up.

At the third floor, the door opens. A kid, chewing gum and sitting on a bicycle, looks at us blankly. "You're going to have to wait," Daniel says. The man starts slipping out the door, and we both grab the board and try to pull him up. The door starts to close, but hits the stretcher and opens again. We push hard against it, and pull up on the stretcher at the same time till it closes.

The elevator descends and opens back on the second floor.

This time we hold the man to prevent him from slipping out. As soon as the door closes, we start CPR again.

Out in the ambulance, we fire more drugs into him, getting a rhythm, but no pulses. By the time we are out at Saint Francis, he is asystole. In the cardiac room, the doctor takes our report, and because the patient is such a young man, continues the effort. They get a rhythm back briefly but again, no pulses. He pronounces him dead.

He thanks us and says we did a good job. And we did. Even though the patient didn't make it, he got great care—our best effort.

Our next call is a priority one chest pain two blocks from the hospital, but the patient turns out to be a fifty-year-old woman with a cold. I feel myself start to say to her, Why did you call us and not just make an appointment with your doctor? but I don't. I can see that she feels awful and doesn't know any better. Because it hurt in her chest when she breathed she thought it might be a heart attack, even though it's the same pain she's been feeling for weeks and she's been coughing up yellow phlegm. She lives here all alone, and maybe seeing someone at the ER will give her some comfort. Maybe I can give her some comfort. I don't argue with her, lecture her, tell her to walk the two blocks, or try to bully her into signing a refusal. I put her on the stretcher, talk nicely to her, and move us along our way so we'll be free for the next call.

The triage nurse has us put her in a wheelchair and we take her to the waiting room. We tell her to listen up for her name being called. She'll probably be seen by a physician assistant in Med-Express where the nonacute patients are seen.

We run into Rebecca again. She is bringing in a patient with CHF. She has the heart monitor over her shoulder and is carrying an IV bag. I help her wheel the man down the hall. She gives a crisp, concise report to the nurse, then puts her hand on the patient's arm and says, "Good luck, Mr. Clark. They'll take good care of you here."

Watching her, I think that I carry with me what others have taught. Now I have passed some of it on.

\* \* \*

Before the day is out, we've done twelve calls, helped twelve people. I sit back at the base catching up on my paperwork when Jackie Lackey, who I turn 471 over to, laughs at my hair, which is all mussed up. "Hard day, huh?" She gets out a camera and starts snapping a picture of me.

I smile. I feel like a medic again. I love my job.

# MEMORY

*I raise my eyes and take in this room, this sight, these people.*

# Joe

He's a double amputee sitting in his bathrobe in an old wheelchair, wearing a World War II army cap. "Shut up, you old witch," he yells at his wife, an old ghostly looking woman in a tattered bathrobe. "You're the one who gave me this damn chest pain."

The apartment is also old, with barely any furniture and a heavy layer of dust over the counters and floor.

"Fifty-two years I've put up with you. Now get out of here and mind your own business."

"Where exactly is the chest pain?" I ask.

"Right here. Like somebody stabbed me. That woman's going to be the death of me."

"Fifty-two years, she must be doing something right," I say as I put a nasal cannula on him to get some oxygen into his system.

My partner has taken the wife into the other room and is getting a list of the medications the patient is on.

"Two years ago she went into the hospital for blood clots. Seventeen months they kept her there. I got used to being a bachelor. Besides, she isn't right in the head anymore. You old witch!" he calls.

"Calm down and breathe easy," I say. His pressure is a little high and his pulse a little fast.

In the ambulance, he says he is feeling better. I have put in a saline lock in case his pressure bottomed out after I gave him a nitro, but since he is feeling better, I now hold off on the nitro.

His heart rhythm is a normal sinus with only a sporadic PVC. I ask him about other medical problems. He says he had a heart attack in 1963, and lost his legs at Guadalcanal in the Pacific.

"I read that book, *Guadalcanal Diary*. That was some battle, huh?"

"Great book," he says. "We chased those nips from the Phillippines to Okinawa. Lost a lot of good men."

"No doubt. You fought for freedom and you won."

"You got that right."

"Feeling better?"

"I think this oxygen is working. And that needle helped too, I suspect."

"Good."

"I know a thing or two about medicine, all the time I spent in the hospital. When I was in the Pacific, there was a woman there at the hospital I was in who gave birth to a kid had three knees."

"Three knees?"

"A right knee, a left knee, and a wee knee," he says.

"That's good," I say.

"I knew a cook there, caught a rare bird, a rhea bird, ever heard of one of those?"

"I think so, sort of like a peacock, isn't it?"

"Yeah. He didn't like the color though, so he decided he'd dye it blue. Guess what happened."

"Tell me."

He tries to keep a straight face but breaks out into a grin. "He got dye-a-rhea."

"That's good. You're killing me."

In the hospital, the staff knows him. "Hey, Joe, how are you today?"

"A little chest pain," he says, "but these fine boys have taken good care of me, feeling much better. We're having a good old time, isn't that right, boys?"

"You got it," I say.

They send us to room ten, bed one.

"First-class accommodations," he says as I wheel him into the empty room.

I am finishing my written report, talking to him as I write, when a nurse comes in to give him a twelve lead EKG.

"EKG," he says, "I had an E-G-G this morning. Does that count for anything?"

"That's a good one," the nurse says.

"I know a thing or two about medicine," he says. "Why, when I was in the hospital in the Pacific, there was a woman who gave birth to a baby with three knees."

Out in the car, I say to Arthur, "As much as I like the medical challenges, I like the people best."

"They can make your day," he says.

"They kill me sometimes."

# Snake Girl

We get called for an insect bite on Capen Street. The apartment is dirty and cluttered. A woman leads us through the living room. I see a cage with a small rabbit in it, munching on a carrot. It looks up at me. Its eyes meet mine as I pass. In the dark hallway there are two small children in diapers, sitting quietly against the wall. I just miss stepping on one. "In here," the woman says.

A woman in her twenties with long, thick hair to her waist sits on the bed, rubbing a spot on her leg. The wound looks like teeth marks. The skin is slightly swollen.

"What bit you?" I ask.

"He bit me," she says. She points to the dresser.

"Holy . . ." I say. There is a huge snake curled up in a glass aquarium.

"He bit me before, but I think some of his teeth are stuck in me this time."

"What kind of snake?"

"He's a boa constrictor. He's been moody lately."

"They're not poisonous, are they? They just like to squeeze things, right?"

"No, they're not poisonous. I think he's hungry. I haven't been feeding him too much. I don't want him getting too big, now that the babies are around. He's over seven feet now. I don't know what I'm going to do with him."

"What does he eat?"

"Rats."

"From around here?"

"No, I get them at the pet store. They cost me three ninety-nine each. He eats fifteen at a time. Hamsters are six dollars. It's getting expensive."

"Is that what the rabbit's for?"

"He wants him. He knows he's out there, that's why he's so wild lately. Getting so I can't take him out."

"You take him out a lot?"

"I take him out every day. We sit outside or walk down the street. He likes it when it's steamy, when the sun comes out bright right after the rain."

"What hospital do you want to go to?"

"Hartford. They took care of me last time."

Coming down the hall, I have to step over the kids again. "Just step on them," the other woman says. "They get out of the way."


"I love snakes ever since I was a little girl," the woman says as we ride to the hospital. "I learned about them in science class. I like their skin and I like the way they hold me. I read about them at night. I know everything about them. I got him when he was just nine inches. Cost me four hundred and fifty dollars. I had to go all the way down to New York City. I got the papers for him."

"When you feed him all those rats, how does he eat them?"

"I dump them all in, and he squeezes them, then he eats them. Takes maybe an hour."

"Do you charge admission when you feed him?"

"No, but I got friends who like to watch."

"What do your kids think about him?"

"They're my sister's kids. I don't got kids."

She is quiet for a while.

"You see that movie *Anaconda*?" I ask.

"Yeah, I was the first one, the first one in line when that come to town. I seen it ten times. I love that movie. It takes place in the jungle. I've read about that place. They got all kinds of animals. I like to go there someday. All the trees and birds. I dream about it at night." Her eyes get a far-off look as she sits there thinking about a place ten thousand miles from the city streets. "Someday I like to have a monkey," she says.


# Polish


We get called for an unknown at Charter Oak Housing, an apartment tower for the elderly. We find a tiny old woman throwing up into a bucket. "No hospital," she says in a thick Polish accident. "No hospital."

The story we get is her daughter, who is an alcoholic, was kicked out of the apartment by the management that morning for being too drunk. Her neighbors are worried the old woman has not been getting enough to eat, and that she is very weak. She has stomach cancer and is very frail.

"No hospital," she says. "No hospital, please."

Joan Dowgielewicz, a new paramedic I am precepting, says for many old Polish people, the hospital is the place they go to die.

She seems alert and oriented, though it is hard to feel a pulse or hear a blood pressure because her arms are bent from osteo-arthritis. I am uncomfortable leaving her, so I decide we are going to take her. "Hospital," I say. "Good place. You go, get better, come home."

"No hospital," she says. "No hospital, please."

We stand her up, and half persuade, half carry her to the stretcher. She does not resist in body. I feel bad about taking her, but this is a case that social service needs to look at.

We wheel her out into the corridor, where her neighbors have gathered. I talk to them briefly, and they express concern for her health, worry that her daughter cannot take care of her.

The patient sees one woman coming out of an apartment door and starts to say something to her in Polish.

"There, there," the neighbor says, brushing the old woman's face.

"You speak Polish?" Arthur asks her.

"Yes."

"Tell her we're going to take her to the hospital, get her checked out, then hopefully she'll be able to come back."

The woman nods, then, looking at the old woman, says very slowly in a loud voice with a pause between each word, "They are going to Take You to the Hospital."

Arthur and I start laughing. She looks at us, offended.

"You said you speak Polish," Arthur says.

"She understands," the woman says defensively. "She understands English."

We try to stop laughing.

"She understands what I was saying. She understands."

"Thank you," Arthur says.

We get in the elevator, shaking our heads.

"She understands," I say.

I look then at the old woman. She sits quietly, her dark eyes peering out of her old wrinkled head. Art pats her on the hand. "You'll be okay," he says.

# Mr. and Mrs. Jones

We're called for an unknown on Vine. The guard asks what apartment we're going to, then he rolls his eyes and says, "They always going at it. He must be drinking again." We knock hard on the door and a young man answers. "My mother called for you," he says.

"Is that the po-lice?" she cries. "Take him out of here. He threatened to kill me."

She is an old woman wearing a Diana Ross wig, sitting in an old armchair.

"What's going on?" I ask.

"He been drinking again. I got asthma and high blood pressure."

A cop arrives and we learn the culprit, her husband, is in the bedroom.

"He ain't taken a bath for months. He give me a venereal disease. I got to take a medication for it. Forty years I been putting up with him. I can't take it no more."

We open the door cautiously and see a man lying in bed, the covers pulled up to his neck. He looks at us as we step in. "What do you want?" he says.

"What's going on?" the cop says.

"Nothing. I'm sleeping."

"You been drinking?"

"Yeah, so what?"

"Your wife says you threatened to kill her."

"I did, 'cause she's been driving me crazy. She never shut up."

"He give me a venereal disease," she shouts.

I can smell the alcohol on his breath.

"Why don't you get up and come with us?"

He throws the sheets off; he is completely naked.

"Where you going to take me?"

I look at the cop and he looks at me. "To the hospital," I say, "So you can sober up and get cleaned up."

"I ain't going nowhere."

"We'll get you something hot to eat," I say.

He looks at me and at the cop, then says, "Now wait a minute. You a white man. I'm naked and this is my own house. Get the fuck out of my house."

"He been drinking all day. Catting about. He ain't never take a bath. And I got asthma," she calls.

"Why don't you put your pants on?" the cop says.

"Get the fuck out of my house," he says. "I don't want no white men in my house when I'm standing here naked. Get the fuck out of my bedroom."

Two other cops arrive. I step back out of the room and let them handle it.

"I got asthma," the woman says, "and he don't give me a minute's sleep when he's been drinking. Forty years I put up with him. No more."

The cops finally convince him to go or be arrested, and while he prefers to be arrested, they prefer he go with me. We take him to Saint Francis, where they put him on a bed in the back hall and restrain him. He's still there the next morning when I come in to work. "How you doing this morning?" I ask.

He doesn't recognize me. He's sober now. "Okay," he says. "Do you know where I could get some orange juice?"


Several months later, we're sent for a difficulty breathing on Bedford Street. A man opens the door and says, "It's my wife, she's got asthma."

"Hey, I know you. Don't you live on Vine?"

"We moved," he says respectfully.

It's the same woman, sitting by the bed. She is in only mild distress. She has some wheezes, so I give her a treatment.

He is on the phone. "Hello, doctor. It's my wife. She's real bad. The ambulance is here. We're going to take her to the hospital. . . . Okay, okay," he says.

"What are you bothering him with?" she says. "Put that phone down and bring me my shoes." She looks at me and shakes her head.

He runs about the house, getting her pocketbook, shoes, and a sweater as we set her on the stretcher and bring her down to the ambulance.

"What a pain in the ass," she says. "Forty years I put up with him."

He hands her her pocketbook. She opens it, takes out an envelope, and removes several twenty-dollar bills, which she stuffs in her bra. "Give this back to him," she says, offering me the envelope.

"He seems to treat you all right," I say.

"He's not so bad, I suppose," she says.

"How you doing, honey?" he calls from the front.

# Memory

In Bellevue Square, we are sent for an infant with a high temperature. As we park in the potholed lot, I notice perhaps sixty or more empty quart-sized bottles lined up in a neat square on a patch of ground between the buildings where only a few strands of grass grow. The sight puzzles me. If someone is collecting bottles, how come they're not in a shopping cart? I put it out of my mind and we go into the building, walk up the graffiti-strewn stairs to the apartment. The husband sits on the couch wearing a bandana around his head and holding a baby. "She ain't eating today and she feel awful hot," he says.

"I know something wrong. I'm trying to take care of her best I can, but I know I had to call for the doctor."

"Where's the baby's mother?"

"She don't live here. She got a drug problem, and I ain't going to have that around my little girl. I set the law on that."

We walk down to the ambulance. My partner points out the bottles to the father.

"My homey got shot there last year."

"Was he dealing drugs?"

"Innocent bystander. We were out there the other night tipping our forties to him."

"Tipping your forties?"

"Drinking beer. I take a drink for myself, then tip some down into the ground for my friend. I know he'd do the same for me. He ain't forgot."

# Where Every Day Is Like Sunday

"I feel like something's pressing against my heart," she says.

Mrs. Mays, an old woman in her seventies, sits in an armchair, her breathing labored.

"Lift up your tongue," I say, placing the small white pill in her mouth. "This will help the pain, and your breathing."

"Thank you," she says.

Arthur comes back with the stair chair we will use to carry her outside and down the creaky front porch steps to our ambulance, parked on this street in the north end of Hartford, where two weeks before we'd done a drug-related shooting.

We are ready to lift her onto our chair when a man comes in the front door and asks the family, "How is she?"

"They just getting ready to take her to Saint Francis. She having trouble with her breathing again."

He is in his fifties, a dark man in a suit and tie. He looks at us. "Do we have time to say a prayer?"

"Go ahead," I say.

They gather hands. Arthur and I step back, but the man says, "Would you like to join us?"

Neither of us are churchgoing, but we step forward and join them. I hold the hand of Mrs. Mays and the hand of her granddaughter, a pretty, modest woman in her thirties.

"We are gathered here in prayer to say thank you, God," the man says. He has a pleasing, humble voice that grows steadily in power. "We offer our blessings for the men who are here to help our sister." He looks at Arthur and me, then bows his head again. "And for the doctors who will soon be helping her. You, Lord, who know all that has come, all that is now, and all that will be, we do not ask why. We do not know the condition or the diagnosis, only you do, but we know that you have your reasons. We thank you for giving us all this great life here, and we hope that we keep on serving you."

"That's right, brother!" the woman holding Arthur's hand calls out.

"Your love for us is strong and we are working hard to be worthy of your kindness."

"Amen!" another woman calls out.

Arthur and I look at each other, then back down at the carpet.

"We hope one day when our labors are done, we will all join you in heaven where every day will be Sunday."

"Tell it, brother!"

"Where *every day* will be Sunday!"

"Yes, sir. Amen!"

"Praise God!"

"We going to keep on working. Going to keep on loving. Keep on striving."

"Sing it out, Deacon!"

"Good God!"

I raise my eyes and take in this room, this sight, these people.

When the prayer is over, there is handshaking and hugging.

"A good prayer, Deacon," the granddaughter says.

"They gone to take good care of her." He nods to us.

"That was a nice prayer," Arthur says. "Thank you."

"God bless you, sister," the deacon says to Mrs. Mays.

"You a good man," she says.

We put her on the chair, wrap her in blankets, and carry her out into the chill, down the creaky gray stairs to where we have the stretcher set up. A kid on a bike with a Walkman on— a lookout—watches us as he circles at the end of the block. Another kid leans against the porch of the house across the street. A pair of sneakers dangle from the telephone wires overhead.

We lift her up on the stretcher. She is heavy, and I can see the strain in Arthur's face, and feel the strain in my back, as we slide her in. I get in with her as Arthur closes the door. I hook her up to the heart monitor. Hers is beating at ninety-two beats a minute with an occasional premature beat, which causes a delay, but the heart waits it out and beats again and picks up its rhythm.

We take her to Saint Francis.

# Reggie and Jill

Reggie Thomas is a regular, a frequent flyer. Nearly every night around eleven we get a call for an intoxicated party on Barber Street. He is either lying on the sidewalk, sitting against a building, or leaning up against a phone booth. He drinks and does heroin. If he is out cold and has pinpoint pupils, we give him Narcan and take him to the ER. If he is just drunk, we help him up into the back of the ambulance and sit him on the bench seat, or let him lie down on it. We take him to Saint Francis. If he is able to open an eye and breathe okay he goes into the crisis unit, where he is strapped down to a bed until he sobers up. If he is really not bad off, he goes into the waiting room, where he watches TV, bums cigarettes, and spends the night, sleeping in a chair, leaving at dawn.

We find him against a street pole. Out of it. Respiratory rate around eight. Pinpoint pupils. I do a sternal rub, and he comes around. "Reggie, buddy, your ride is here."

He grunts, but we lift him up. He can barely put his feet under him. "Looks like a Narcan night," I say to my partner.

"No!" Reggie screams. He swings his arms to break free. "Don't give me that Narcan shit. Cuz! Cuz! They going to give me that Narcan. Help me, brother. I spent my last twenty dollars!"

"Easy, easy," I say. "We're just going to check you out first. If you can stay awake, we won't give it to you."

"No, man, not that shit."

We get him in the back, and he starts nodding off. I nudge him awake. "Don't give me that Narcan shit," he says.

"Look, you're breathing semi-okay. I'll make a deal with you. You let me put an IV in your arm. I won't give you the Narcan unless you completely go out on me. Okay?"

He grunts and sticks his arm out for me.

After I am done with the IV, he falls asleep. His vitals are okay. His respirations are about twelve. He just needs watching.

At Saint Francis, I explain the story. He's been doing heroin, but I didn't give him any Narcan. He is right on the edge. Needs watching but should be okay. They put him in the crisis unit.

When I come back with the paperwork, he is lying in bed, one eye open. He recognizes me, and says, "Come here, man." He takes my hand. "You treat me all right. I love you, man." He kisses my hand. "I love you."

I pick him up again the next night. "I just have to check your pupils," I say once we get him in the back. He lays his head down on the bench seat. His pupils are pinpoint.

"You been doing heroin again?"

"Every damn day," he says.

"You been drinking?"

"Every damn day."

"I don't think you need any Narcan tonight."

He sits up quickly. "Don't give me that."

"No, no, I'm not going to. I was just saying you didn't need any Narcan."

"Don't say that word, man." He puts his hands over his ears. "Don't say that word."

They put him in a wheelchair and park him across from the triage desk. He dozes off. "Watch this," I say to Rachelle Mastroninizio, the triage nurse. I nod to my partner, Mark Rozyn, who goes behind Reggie and whispers in his ear. We wait. Five seconds pass. Ten seconds. Then suddenly, he shudders so hard the blanket falls off him. A nightmare passes and he drifts back to sleep.

"What did he say to him?" Rachelle asks.

"Narcan," I say. "The word is like kryptonite to him."

It's the night of the NCAA basketball finals. Fifteen minutes to tipoff. I'm standing in the Saint Francis waiting room watching the pregame commentary. It's been a slow night. I'm hoping I'll be able to watch a good part of the game, but then the portable goes off. "Four-seven-one, Westland and Barber for an intoxicated party."

When we get there Reggie is lying on the ground.

Over the PA, I say, "Reggie Thomas, your ride is here. Please stand, and move to the corner."

I see him lift his head slightly, but he doesn't get up.

I get out and stand over him. He gets up and smiles. "Hey, man," he says. "Do I have alcohol on my breath?" He blows at me.

"A little bit," I say.

"Take me to Saint Francis."

"But of course."

"Let me just grab my dinner." He goes over to the pay phone where he has a Styrofoam food cartoon resting on the ground. "Let's go," he says.

In the ambulance, he is animated, more alert than I've seen him in weeks.

At Saint Francis he tells the triage nurse he's okay, the waiting room will be fine tonight. He glances at my watch. "Can you get me some ginger ale?" he asks me. "I know you're my buddy."

I get him a small can from the kitchen. I find him parked under the TV, looking up at the screen. Just in time for the opening tip. "Kentucky all the way," he says. His container, open on his lap, is filled with ribs and fries.

At four in the morning, I look in the waiting room, and see him slumped in a chair, sound asleep, his head resting on the head of another regular, who wears a Kentucky T-shirt over his dirty jacket. His head is on Reggie's shoulder.

At five in the morning, Joe Stefano responds to a call for a drunk on Albany Avenue and discovers Reggie leaning against the phone. "Where the hell have you been and what the hell are you doing here?" Joe demands.

Reggie looks at him through his heroin-and-booze-glossed eyes like he is a crazy man. "What you talking about, man?"

"You're out of the neighborhood, and do you know what time it is?"

"Huh?"

"It's five o'clock in the damn morning. Do you know how worried we have been? You were supposed to call at eleven. When you didn't call by midnight, we started getting concerned, and you've had us worried to death for the last several hours wondering where the hell you are. For all we know you could have been dead."

"Sorry, man, I didn't know."

"If you're going to be out of the neighborhood and staying out to all hours, do us the courtesy and let us know."

"Okay, man, sorry."

"Don't let it happen again."

"I didn't know you kept track."

"I ought to give you some Narcan just to teach you a lesson."

"No, no not that."

"We have an understanding, then?"

"I'll call next time."

"Home to Saint Francis?"

"Home to Saint Francis," he says. "You okay, man."

Jill Abott is ten days older than me, and I think she wouldn't be bad looking if she hadn't spent the last ten years of her life on the street. I pick her up one day passed out in front of the Bradlees store off Park. She has vomit in her hair and her face is blue. She has an empty bottle of antiseptic by her side. At first I think she isn't breathing. I reposition her airway, and put her on 100 percent oxygen. Her color improves, but she is completely unresponsive. Ammonia inhalants don't work, sternal rubs. Nothing. I take her to Hartford Hospital, and six hours later I see her back out on the street walking into a liquor store.

I'm working a night shift. It's past midnight when she comes up to the ambulance and flashes me one of her smiles.

"Jill," I say. "I heard you were dead."

She laughs. "No, not me. I got another birthday coming up. Though Jack Garza died last week. He was only twenty-eight. And Manny Gonzales is dead. I found him behind the liquor store on High Street and called the cops. I'm hoping to make my next birthday."

"I'm sure you will," I say.

"I'm not drinking no more," she says. "Could you lend me some money so I can get some coffee? I've been being real good. I got to make that birthday. It's hard, you know, it's hard. I stay sober for a while, then I take a fall, but I'm going to do it, I'm working real hard this time. Please lend me some money so I can get a cup of coffee and maybe something to eat."

I give her sixty-one cents, all the change in my pocket.

"Thanks, you're great. I won't forget your kindness."

Ten minutes later I go into the Shell convenience market on Capitol and Broad, and Jill is standing at the counter with change spread out and a bottle of Listerine on the counter. "Hey, Peter," she says. "Can you lend me forty cents so I can make a purchase?"

I look at the Listerine. "No, I'm not going to give it to you so you can drink the mouthwash, and I'll have to pick you up later. I thought you said you'd quit."

She smiles. "I got a sore throat. A real bad one."

"Yeah, right."

"I need to gargle."

The cashier takes the Listerine off the counter.

"How about buying me a cup of coffee?" she says.

Four hours later, I see her at Hartford Hospital in the drunk station, where she is strapped into a wheelchair. "So you got your Listerine after all," I say.

"It was for my throat," she says. "I had a hankering for it."

"Nice breath," I say.

She laughs and smiles. She looks just like a little girl.

# You Ain't Fooling Me

The family has called because their great-grandmother is acting crazy and they want her taken away. She is close to ninety and sits in an armchair by the door with her walker in front of her. She isn't budging. "Please don't take me away," she says. "I ain't crazy. I ain't crazy. Lord help me, I ain't crazy."

"She has a point," Arthur says. "She knows where she is and there is nothing physically wrong with her. We can't take her without papers."

I have tried to persuade her but to no avail. "I been to a nursing home before," she says, "when I broke my hip, and they nice people, real nice, but I ain't going. You can't make me."

I confer with the family. "We really can't take her. It would be kidnapping. If you want her put in a home, you'll have to work with social services."

"But they said that can take a month."

"We can't take her. Like I said, it would be kidnapping."

I go out to the car to get a refusal for her to sign, but when she sees me coming with the paper, she gets up and starts moving away from me, a walker step at a time. "I ain't signing that," she says. "You ain't fooling me. I may be old, but I'm no fool. I ain't signing that. Lord help me. I ain't signing that. You ain't fooling me. You ain't fooling me."

I stand there with the refusal in my hand as she makes her slow escape.


# There Must Be a Mistake


We're taking a ninety-year-old woman to Saint Francis to have her hip looked at. Arthur is teching the call. "Why, there must be some mistake," he says. "This paperwork says you were born in 1907, but that would make you ninety years old and you don't look a day over seventy-five."

"Oh, you are so kind," the woman says, "but I'm ninety."

"No," Arthur says. He calls to me, "Peter, how old do you think this nice lady is?"

"Not a day over seventy-five," I say.

"It says here, she's ninety years old."

"There must be some mistake," I say. "That couldn't be."

"It must be a mistake," Arthur says. "I don't believe it. You're much too young-looking."

"Oh, you boys," she says.

*  *  *

Arthur sits in back with a lady we're returning to her nursing home after a two-week hospital stay. Arthur reads the discharge summary, which describes the woman as a "pleasantly confused eighty-year-old."

"Pleasantly confused, a nice term," he says.

"Where are you taking me?" the woman asks.

"Back to the nursing home."

"Have I been there before?"

"Yes, you liked it very much."

"How nice," she says.

"And where are we going?" she asks later.

"To the nursing home."

"Oh, very good. I've heard it's very nice. Have I been there before?"

"Pleasantly confused," Arthur says after we've left her. "That's what I'd like to be."

"You're not far from it," I say.

"What?"

"Hard of hearing, too."

"There must be some mistake," Arthur says to the eighty-eight-year-old lady riding in back with him as he reads her hospital discharge papers. "It says there, you were born in 1909. That would make you eighty-eight, when you can't be a day over seventy-five."

"Oh, yes, I'm eighty-eight."

"I don't believe it. Hey, Peter, how old do you think this lady is?"

"Not a day over seventy-five."

"It says here she's eighty-eight. It must be a typo."

"Has to be a typo. She doesn't look a day over seventy-five."

"Must be a mistake," Arthur says.

"No, I'm eighty-eight," she says.

"I don't believe it," Arthur says.

On the way out of the nursing home, Arthur says he's got to take a pee. He looks around for a restroom. "Take a right at the corner," I say.

"How do you know?"

"It's what the sign says right there." I point to it.

He studies the sign a moment, then says, "I'll be damned."

I wheel the stretcher out by myself and am remaking it when he emerges.

"You know," I say, "I was just thinking that one of these days we're going to go in together, and I'm going to come out by myself."

"Hey," he says.

"Yup, we'll get a call to go to the nursing home, but they won't give us a name to pick up, and while they strap you to your wheelchair and give you a tray of macaroni and diced peaches, you'll be crying, 'There must be some mistake.' I'll be coming out by myself, wiping a solitary tear from my eye."

"Well, if I'm pleasantly confused, then I guess it won't matter."

We lift the stretcher up together and throw it in back.

"The years, they do go by," I say.

"Enough of that," he says.

# Right There

She is ninety-three years old. She lives in a small, well-ordered room in a residential development for the elderly. She weighs barely eighty pounds. Her face is deeply wrinkled. She says she used to be a dancer—that is her secret to living so long. She tells me how she met her husband at the bar where she worked, and how, on their fiftieth anniversary, she got up on the table and did a tap dance that brought the house down. She has an easy laugh and asks me about my own life, the ladies I have known.

She is going to the hospital because she has a pain in her side when she breathes. I ask her where it is exactly. She takes my hand, brings it around her back, moving it up her ribs, to feel the place. I can feel her delicate carriage. She presses my hand against the spot. Suddenly she arches her back and cries out in a quick gasp.

"Right there," she says.

"Right there," I say.

Her skin is warm. She keeps my hand against her back. I can feel her breathe. I can feel myself breathe. It is quiet. She smiles at me softly. In her eyes, I see her twenty-year-old self, sitting close to me in the evening. I see the eyes of all the women I have loved. I think growing old may not be all that bad.


# Flirt


We are in triage at Mount Sinai with a forty-year-old woman who has been hearing voices most of her life. Jack and Diane are the ones talking to her today. "They always in my bidness," she tells me. We picked her up at the community health center, where the doctor said she needed to get her medications stabilized. Though she is forty, she looks much younger, with a soft, freckled brown baby face. She has no teeth. I have told her that she looks familiar to me and I speculated that I may have picked her up before. She doesn't remember me and the more I look at her, the more I think she looks like my friend Kevin Andrews, who has about ten brothers and sisters, and many more cousins.

"Do you have a brother named Kevin?" I ask.

"No."

"You look like this guy I know."

"I don't know, maybe I do. I may have more brothers and sisters than I know about."

"How's that?"

"My mother only had eleven kids," she tells me.

"Only eleven?"

"Yeah, but my father had nineteen that he know about."

"Nineteen!"

"So maybe if there's one unaccounted for, maybe I might have a brother named Kevin. I don't know."

"Nineteen. Is he still out there putting them out?"

"No, he's a paraplegic. He fell off a ladder a few years ago."

"Oh, I'm sorry."

"No, don't be. He get around good. He got one of them carts."

"That's good, I guess."

She smiles a beautiful toothless smile. "He still flirt," she says.

# THE JOB

*This is still the best job on earth because we get to do what we love: answer calls. . . . It's just my partner and me and the patient. And we do what we are good at. Help people.*

# Thanks

Arthur and I are sitting in our ambulance in a park across town, while we wait for our number to be called. Arthur reads the paper. I watch the young mothers play with their kids on the swing sets. "So the head of EMS resigned," he says. "I thought you saved his job."

"We did," I say. "But they took his responsibilities away and gave him a broom and told him to sweep all day. He had enough, so he quit in protest."

Arthur grunts.

"There's an editorial in there about it," I say.

He turns to the page I point out. It's titled: HEALTH COMMISSIONER'S END RUN?

He reads part of it aloud. The gist of it is, despite the fact that our rally at the capitol convinced the legislature to stop the budget cuts, the health commissioner has gone ahead and dismantled the Office of Emergency Medical Services through other means, prompting the resignations of the EMS head and his second in command.

"The commissioner shouldn't be allowed to abuse his power like that."

"It'll come back to haunt him. I have no doubt he'll get his. In the meantime people will suffer."

Arthur shakes his head. "Typical government."

"Tell me about it."

The Commissioner may have gotten what he wanted today, but he has set himself up for a fall. Someday someone important is going to die and, rightly or wrongly, people will question whether or not the EMS system failed them. There'll be newspaper headlines, public outcry, and investigations. The legislature will react as they often do, making dramatic, but not always well-thought-out changes, when what is needed now is calm deliberation and forethought. Fix the system today, don't wait until the disaster to react.

I am disappointed by what has happened at the state. I thought we had done something great and succeeded beyond our expectations, but while a citizen can stand up and be heard, unless you have power on the inside looking out for your interests—keeping your gains is another story.

Across the field, I notice an older couple walking hand in hand, coming our way, and the sight cheers me a little. Isn't that nice. In our job you see so much sickness and dying, it is good to see people happy, people healthy. The couple nears, and I notice they are looking at us, actually coming up to talk to us.

"You remember me," the man says.

"No, I don't," I say, but to keep them from feeling bad, I say, "You look familiar."

"You came and got me on Prospect Avenue when I was having my heart attack."

"You boys saved my Fred's life," his wife says.

"Oh, yeah, I remember now," I say. "How are you?"

"Doing great. Out walking every day."

"You look well." Arthur says.

"He was in the hospital for two months. But he's home now and doing great, aren't you, Fred?"

"Never better," he says.

"Isn't that nice. That's great."

"Thanks again," he says.

"God bless you both," the woman says.

They wave and walk off, still hand in hand.

"Remember him?" I ask.

"No."

"Me, neither."

"They remembered us."

"I guess that's not hard to do. A big guy like you."

"And an old man like you."

"That's something we don't hear every day."

"Yeah, it was almost out of TV land. Amazing."

"I was thinking the same thing."

"Except where were the TV cameras and the picnic spread? They always get a picnic on TV."

"You can't have everything."

"I know."

"Nice couple."

I look up the call later that night. I keep copies of all the run forms I have done, thousands. At first every name meant something to me, now they are all a blur: chest pains, diabetics, strokes, motor vehicle accidents, cardiac arrests. At least I have the address to go on. I find it. The run form is shorthand, abbreviations.

67 y/o male with crushing substernal chest pain x half an hour. Onset while at rest with diaphoresis and nausea. Prior history MI, HTN. A-0X3, skin, pale, cool, clammy. Anxious. Positive JVD, rales in bases, ab soft non-tender, pedal edema. BP-102/56 P-96 R-28, Pulse Sat-92%. Sinus with ST elevation in Leads II and III and multifocal PVCs.

O2 at 15 lpm via nonrebreather. IV # 18 in L FA Saline Lock. 162 mg ASA PO. 80 mg Lasix IVP. .4 mg NTG SL. Extricated via stair chair.

Medical control contacted. Orders received for additional 40 mg Lasix IVP and 4 mg MS IVP provided pressure stays above 90 systolic. 2nd IV # 16 in R AC NS KVO.

PVCs diminished with O2. Meds given as above. Vitals reaccessed. Substernal pressure slightly improved after 2nd .4 mg NTG and 4 mg MS IVP. Lungs improved post Lasix. Pt calmer. Still some pressure in chest. SAT 99% with O2. Vitals on arrival BP 100/60 P-88 R-22.

Taken priority one and turned over to ER staff with full report.

Words on paper. They don't convey the fear in their eyes, the touch of our hands, the whirl of minutes, the beat of hearts. For so many of our calls we never find out what happens, unless we read their names in the obits. It can give us a tough slant on the job. It is a good lesson to remember the ones we help, even if we won't recognize them on the street. I think about the file cabinets I have filled, the thousands of sheets of paper, all that medical terminology—the record of what I have done. They are not just forms, but people who walk the earth, and whom we were there for in their moments of crisis. It is so easy in this job to forget the basics of what we do and how much we help people. They, the patients, the people, they are what makes it all worthwhile. They are who we have to remember when we find our spirits lagging. They are what it is all about, from the one-on-one contact between paramedic and patient to the efficient running of the entire EMS system. They are what we fight for. They are what makes it worthwhile.

# Exeter

My friend Brad finally drags me to Exeter, the prep school we attended, for the annual football game with the school's archrival, Andover. He says I owe him for not going to our twentieth reunion. I had wimped out at the last minute, not wanting to go back to the school I had hated, where I had struggled constantly, never feeling that I met its standards. When Brad is badgering me to go, I tell him I have three conditions—one, that we have a designated driver as I will need alcohol to fortify me; two, that if I choose not to set foot on the campus, he cannot make me, and will have to meet me at a bar after the game; and three, that he hound me daily until the day arrives, as I am apt to back out from fear of returning. He agrees to all three conditions.

Shortly after I park my car in his driveway, our driver arrives and takes us up there. "Feeling it in the pit of your stomach?" Brad asks as we hit the town limits.

"Not yet," I say tensely.

Our driver lets us off by the academy building, a huge ivied and marble brick building where we took most of our classes and sat in thrice-weekly assemblies in the giant hall. As we walk through the campus and out to the athletic field, I feel oddly detached. It is like I am walking through the set of an old movie I only vaguely remember. I am not the person now that I was then.

We walk over the river and take our seats in the stadium, the stone coliseum. Brad played football here; this is the first time I have even been to the stadium. It is cold and windy. The football team is terrible and we leave at half-time with the score Andover 21, Exeter 0.

We go to a bar in town and drink pitchers of beer and talk. I tell Brad about my big playoff hit in my last softball game of the year—a bases-clearing triple to tie the score with two outs in the bottom of the last inning. "Winter was coming down," I say. "Then the pitch came in. The second baseman broke for the middle, anticipating my predictable drive over second, but I saw him move out of the corner of my eye. I shifted my shoulder slightly and drove the ball right to where he had just been—a cruise missile that gapped the outfielders all the way to the fence as I ran around the bases, ran like the wind, like Mercury, like a man chased by wolves."

"Did you win?"

"No, I got stranded, then pitching, I gave up six runs in the top of the first extra inning, and we lost by six."

"So you weren't really the hero."

"No, but I almost was."

Brad has had a hard go of it lately. He lost his election for county sheriff in the Democratic landslide. Boston newspapers headlined his opponent's smear campaign claiming that Brad left the county bankrupt, in spite of Brad's vehement denial. Months later when an auditor's report cleared him, there was only a small article in the *Boston Herald*, and not a word in the *Boston Globe*, which had run a photo of his opponent holding a shredder. Politics is a dirty business, he has learned, but he wants to keep at it, despite a large personal campaign debt he is struggling to pay off. He wants to prove you can be an honest person and an effective officeholder. We talk about other things as well. His oldest boy, William, is turning into quite a good hockey player. His daughters, Liza and Catherine, love soccer, and his youngest, Charles, is just starting hockey. He loves his wife, Susan; their marriage is strong and she has stood by him through his two heartbreaking election losses.

I think of the letter I received from our close classmate Brad Lown, who was one of our most gifted athletes, now a lawyer in New Hampshire, who himself had run for public office in his state. He wrote about Brad Bailey, "He, as do you and I, hankers to be a big shot someday, and maybe he will be in some sense. But as I have gotten older the allure of being a big shot has waned, and I'm not sure that being a good father, husband, and an honest lawyer isn't the very best way to make my mark on the world."

When we leave the bar, we go to a market and buy a six-pack of tallboys—the same market we'd buy beer from, or think about buying beer from, when we were students. It is dark and we wander about the campus. I head off by myself to my old dorm, and stand outside in the darkness looking for a glimpse of my old self in the window, studying at my desk, sitting in a chair reading a history assignment, or just lying on my bed, looking up at the ceiling, dreaming. But I am no longer there.

We meet in the academy building and go up to sit in the great assembly hall. I find the portrait of William Ernest Gillespie in the back with the inscription from his commencement address in June 1967. It reads: "It is nearly time for you to be off, you have a lot to do. This is no time to concern yourselves with nostalgia. As a matter of fact I don't believe anybody has ever claimed that Exeter is a warm nest, but I hope and I expect that when you find yourselves involved in skirmishes, on the frontiers of barbarism, which are not very far away, you'll strike some shrewd blows in favor of civilization. Some day you'll come back to show us your trophies and your scars, and we'll be glad to see you."

The word "shrewd" I hadn't remembered. I believe Brad and I have struck blows, but they haven't been shrewd blows, anything but. More like blind thrusts. We have our scars, our struggles are written in the lines of our faces and in the hidden sorrows of our hearts, but we have survived.

We sit in the back of the empty hall, raise our beers and toast the boys we were then and the men we are now.

"Father," I say to Brad, "husband, friend, public servant, Red Sox fan."

"Paramedic," he says to me.

"Softball hero," I add.

"Legend in your own mind," he says.

"Legend nonetheless," I say.

When we leave, we walk down the marble stairs, and startle a janitor who is locking up. I momentarily think to hide the beer can in my hand, but then don't. "We were just revisiting old times," I say to the man. "Reminiscing."

He growls and points out the side exit, which he hasn't locked yet.

Outside we raise our beers again, one last time. "Here's how they do it in Hartford," I say. And we take a drink, then tip our "forties," pouring the beer into the earth to share it with our ghosts, our memories.

Our ride is waiting in the driveway and we head home, back to our lives.

# Asthma

We're two blocks away from the call when HPD dispatches us to a difficulty-breathing asthma on Martin Street. The woman meets us at the curb. She is leaning against the fence, unable to

move. I can see the panic in her eyes. I unwrap my stethoscope
from around my neck and listen to her lungs as she holds herself up. No air movement. Nothing. Nada. I shout at Arthur to
pull the stretcher. We set her on it and quickly lift her into the
back. "Ever been intubated before?" I ask. She nods fearfully.
She is using all her accessory muscles to breathe. Arthur is
putting a treatment together. She reads 64 on the pulse SAT.
Pulse of 140. I don't even try for a blood pressure. I am immediately on the mike to the hospital asking for medical control.

"Approximately thirty-year-old female, history asthma, including intubation, no audible air movement at this time, really
straining, pulse one-forty, SAT sixty-four, giving her a treatment, would like orders for point-three milligrams epi SQ."

The standard practice is at least two treatments before the
epi, but the treatments aren't going to get it done. As I'm
talking to the doctor, her respirations seem to be slowing. She
is exhausted, on the verge of respiratory arrest.

"Go ahead," the doctor says.

I flip open the biotech and reach for a one cc syringe and an
ampule of epi. "Get out the thing," I say to Arthur. I break the
glass ampule with an alcohol wipe, draw up .3 cc.

"Here's the thing," Arthur says, laying the ambu-bag on the
bench along with my airway kit.

I jab the needle into the woman's arm on an angle and push it
in. "This should help," I say.

She is no longer focusing. I fear I am losing her. I reach for
my intubation kit. I unzip it, take out a 7.0 tube, and the number-
three MacIntosh blade, which I snap into the laryngoscope.
She is turning blue. I will not fail this time. I will not fail. "I'm
going to put it in your throat," I say, spreading her teeth apart.
She is going out on me. I thrust the blade in and sweep her
tongue out of the way. The light illuminates her throat. Her
arms come up as she starts to gag. I get a glimpse of the cords
straining for air. I push the tube down her throat. I'm in. Arthur
hands me the bag and I attach it to the tube and start ventilating. The air goes in. I see her chest rise. "Easy, easy," I say.
Suddenly she is reaching for the tube, fighting against the foreign object in her throat.

I try to hold the tube, and block her arms with my elbows. Arthur grabs her arms. "Easy, easy." Her eyes are open, looking about wildly. "Let me breathe for you. I'm breathing for you." Sweat from my forehead lands on hers. Her color is coming back. "Let me breathe for you," I say.

Her eyes are fixed on me now. "Are you okay?"

She nods.

"I had to do this, you were going out."

She nods.

"I didn't want to lose you. We've got to keep the tube in there for now."

I keep squeezing the bag, synchronizing the squeezes with her own efforts to breathe. We breathe as one. On the pulse oximeter now she is up to 99 percent. The epi is in and now with the tube forcing air into her lungs, we're getting the job done.

Arthur takes us to the hospital.

"For a minute, I thought it was Nicki Joyner all over again," I say to Arthur as we walk back out to the ambulance.

"But we were there this time," he says.

"Yes, we were. By the way, thanks for getting the thing out." He pats me on the back. "My pleasure," he says.

In the ER, they give the woman several breathing treatments down the tube, IV fluid, and steroids. They will keep her in the hospital for a couple days, then she will go home to her family.

Later, driving through the city, I think there are days when the city seems sharper, more colorful. You see people's faces, their individual smiles. Amid the din of sounds, you hear human voices, laughter. You feel a part of the life.

"You all right?" Arthur asks.

"Yes, I am, I'm fine," I say.

# Change

The company gives us a new schedule. Instead of three twelve-hour shifts, we are all to work two twelve-hour shifts and two eights. That means another fifty-two days of the year I have to go to work. We rebid the schedule. Partners who have worked together for years are broken up. I lose my shift with Arthur and end up moving to nights.

When I started in EMS I worked for a small mom-and-pop commercial ambulance service in Springfield, Massachusetts. Eastern Ambulance's home base was a far cry from the fire station that had housed the *Emergency* paramedics on TV. In the garage was a dusty Fleetwood ambulance that hadn't seen the road for decades and three other junked rigs, whose parts had been cannibalized to keep the rest of the fleet running. Off the garage was a dimly lit rec room with a pool table that cost you two quarters to use, moth-eaten couches, paperback books from the fifties, a Coke machine with an out-of-order sign on it, and a windowless sleeping room with squeaky wire cots. The place looked more like the set from *Taxi*.

The pay was terrible. I started at $5.50 an hour and worked up to $6.00 after three months. The highest pay rate was $8.00 an hour. Many people hadn't had a raise in three or four years. The equipment was poor, too. The in-house suction on the ambulance was unreliable and our wooden backboards were splintering. I don't know how many times car 7 would cut out on us when we were en route with full lights and sirens. We'd kick it into neutral, turn the ignition again, and continue on our way.

The shocks were bad. Sometimes the brakes or steering got so bad in one of the rigs, we would refuse to drive it. A shift didn't seem to go by without one of the rigs going down to Robbie's garage for repairs. Originally we had two backup rigs, then one, then none. Sometimes we'd work a crew short. Our owner made vague promises about new ambulances, but they never materialized. Neither did the raises. In many respects the ambulance company was a disgrace to EMS.

But the employees were loyal. It was a family-run business and that atmosphere helped. If you needed time off, you got it. If your phone rang at six-thirty Sunday morning and Lynn Delaney, the dispatcher, asked you in her sweet Southern voice if you could possibly fill in for the next twenty-four hours, you said yes because you knew they'd help you out when you needed time off. Some techs had been there nine and ten years, working seventy-two or more hours a week. You got attached to the people. They helped you—taught you to be a good EMT. Doing calls together—whether a bad MVA or watching the progression of a regular cancer chemotherapy patient—bound you together. Steve, M. J., Christine, Abdullah, David, Kevin, Brian, Sherry, Linda, Bob—these and others were my teachers.

In time, I learned how to drive like a chauffeur, taking care to ease the bumps and go smooth on the turns. In the back I learned how to take a blood pressure and pulse despite the rough road and sirens, and how to write the run report without scrawling all over the page. And I learned how to treat people decently from watching the EMTs around me. Abdullah, the manager, stressed patient care and we took pride in that even when we couldn't take pride in our equipment. It was the people and their attitudes that made the place.

We lost one of our 911 contracts to another company, who offered defibrillation and paramedic intercepts. The company owner was ill and his wife was doing her best just to keep the place running, much less put money back into it in such hard times. With the bad Northeastern economy, with many people without insurance, and with Medicare and Medicaid paying only a portion of the bill when they paid at all, the till was running dry. Fifty percent of the accounts were uncollected. Soon we went down to three crews, then two after five at night.

Then we heard the company was calling it quits. I worked my last shift on a rainy Sunday, with Steve Czyprena. Driving around one of the towns we covered, he pointed out the intersections where he had worked MVAs and the houses he'd taken people out of. "People know me in this town," he said. "They don't know my name, but they recognize me. I felt a part of things here."

Eastern was a big family. People feuded with each other, bitched about equipment and living conditions, and griped about the pay, but they stuck together. Closing down was hard. Some of the younger ones got hired right away by the competition. Most of the older techs needed more time to think about their alternatives. You don't go into this field for money and there's no real future in it. Ten years in one place, then you're out of a job. No more climbing into the same old rig, spending seventy-two hours a week with the same partner, responding to calls for help at all hours of the day and night, all for eight bucks an hour. It's a hard business. It gets in your blood and won't let go.


Today most of those people are still in EMS and working in various locations for the same big company that I work for. It is a different feeling. There are some pros to it—the equipment is top of the line, the cars well maintained. But it is a business, which is the bottom line with commercial EMS. It exists to make profit. Our union negotiates a contract that fails to keep up with the cost of living, and significantly lowers pay for all future employees. Our negotiators tell us it is the best they can do. The company, operating on orders from corporate headquarters, says they can't and won't offer more. We vote the contract down by a huge majority. What will it lead to? A better contract? Impasse? A strike? Large-scale firings? A busted union? All of us working for even less? Or the division closed down and all of us going to work for the competition, losing all seniority, making less money?

I read where an ambulance executive of another corporation

allegedly said in a meeting that if a paramedic owns a house, he is making too much money. I picture a corporate meeting where they go over company finance reports and earnings projections. Cut cars, cut personnel, give us that big dividend. I try to picture an alternative, where the executive says to the paramedic, "You've worked hard, you're stressed out after that dead baby call, take six months off, and here's a five grand bonus so you and the wife can go to Hawaii." It's not long till that company goes bankrupt. I know capitalism has its rules. The lines on the charts need to go up, not down. I understand that. Maybe we should be thankful we have jobs. There are paramedic classes churning out new medics more than happy to take our places. Meat in the seat.

It is too easy to blame the corporate bosses. They are filling a need. Towns and cities are trying to cut costs. Most pay big bucks for police and fire. It doesn't leave much for the new kid on the block, EMS. Why pay salaries and pensions for paramedics when a commercial company will provide the service for next to nothing, or, in the case of Hartford (or other big cities with a sufficient call volume to support the business), for free? What do taxpayers care if after twenty years of working side-by-side on dangerous calls, the police officer and firefighter get generous pensions when the paramedic gets nothing? Spit. Shown the door with broken back and spirit. The smart ones, those who started young enough, leave to work for fire or police departments. Shawn Kinkade gets hired by East Hartford Fire. Mike Lambert goes to Manchester Fire. Tom Harper gets a job as a construction foreman. Shirley Lessard goes back to running a hair salon. Kelly Tierney becomes an insurance adjuster. Others leave the field for "real jobs"—selling, nursing, truck driving.

I admit to being discouraged. I don't like to think of myself as replaceable, although we all are. I don't like having to work four days a week, and being in a different car with a different set of gear every night, and I am not crazy about the corporate logo on the back of my jacket. I bitch along with everyone else, and all the bitching does is wear me down.

The truth is I love what I do. So do my coworkers. We all could do something else and make more money, but we don't. We love our jobs. The years start to go by, opportunities for some slip past, but many stay because for all the bullshit, this is still the best job on earth because we get to do what we love. Answer calls. And on the call, the ambulance service, the logo, the pension or lack of it, the pay make no difference. It's just my partner and me and the patient. And we do what we are good at. Help people.

One night after the new schedules have begun, I see Missy Young washing the windows of her ambulance outside Saint Francis.

"With the way these cars have been getting beat to hell lately, your car is looking like the prize of the fleet," I say. My car, like others, is trashed. Not having regular cars, some of the pride has gone out of it. The cars are not getting washed, checked, and stocked like they used to.

"I don't care that I have to clean a new one every night," she says. "This is my home for the next twelve hours, and I want my patients to feel comfortable here, like they were in my own home."

I look at my ambulance, the dirt caked on the sides. Winter weather is hard on it. If I wash it now, I probably will have to wash it again in a couple hours, so why bother, I say to myself. But Missy is right, of course, though it takes me a couple days to come around to it. I get tired of looking at the dirt, tired of listening to the complaining, others' and my own. This is my car. My work. My patient. My professional care. I pull the car I am assigned into the garage bay and park it by the hose. I turn the water on and start hosing it down. I dip the broom into a bucket of soapy water, then start scrubbing the sides, scrubbing hard. I wash the ambulance. I wash it till it gleams.

# Ups and Downs

I'm sitting at the office talking to Rick Domina, who I think is one of the best medics in the company. We're talking about burnout. It is true that some people stay on the job too long, become jaded, incapable of feeling, and stop caring altogether. But he says that for him—and for many medics that he has known—the longer he works at this job, the more temperate his feelings. When you start, the highs are really high, and the lows are very low. Everyone goes through periods of burnout. Sometimes it seems you'll never get out, but if you make it through the bad ones, you get better. At least for him, that's proved true. The bumps are less abrupt, and the emotional line straightens, but it isn't flat. It has little regular blips. Like life.

I hope that is how it works out for me.

# Last Day Together

I will miss Arthur. We fought, but we had good times and came to an understanding. He went a little easier on the air horn; I gave him a little more time to wash his hands and use the bathroom between calls.

I tell him I finally figured a way to get rid of him—conspire with a large national corporation to take over our company and change the shifts.

He laughs. "You're going to miss me," he says.

"I won't miss you," I say. "I won't miss you at all."

Arthur is paired with Rick Ortyl. I joke that I have traded him for a Snickers bar, but I only get a minisized bar. I point this out to Arthur. "Depreciation," I say. "I got you from Shawn for a regular-sized bar."

"It's 'cause you wore me down," he says.

On our last day together, they send us out to Windsor for a woman going into the hospital for cellulitis. "Let us know if you need a lift assist when you get there," the dispatcher says.

Arthur and I have never called for a lift assist in our two years of working together. But when we enter the woman's apartment, we understand what the dispatcher was talking about. She is nearly five hundred pounds. Fortunately, she is able to stand herself with the help of her motorized pivot chair, and we have our one-man stretcher that means if we can get her on it, then lift the stretcher part up while keeping the wheels on the ground, we ought to be able to slide the stretcher into the ambulance. "We can do this," I say.

She stands and we get her to lie down on the stretcher, then roll her outside in the down position. We bend our knees. I pull the trip, and we drive up with our legs. Upright. We slide the top of the stretcher in the ambulance, then I lift up, keeping my back straight, and Arthur brings the wheels up, and we're in. Done. Good work.

When Rebecca sees us wheeling our patient into Hartford Hospital, she asks if we lifted her ourselves. She says when she was sent for the same patient, she had to call for the fire department, who carried the woman out in a Stokes basket. "We did her ourselves," I say. "Just solid lifting technique and brute animal strength."

"With a couple ibuprofen thrown in," Arthur says.

"You guys are too much," she says.

"The last of a dying breed," I say.

* * *

We respond on a priority one for an unconscious person. The man is cold, clammy, and has poor respirations. He is a diabetic. Arthur assists his respirations with an ambu-bag while I get the IV. His blood sugar is 0. I give him an amp of D50 and he wakes up. His breathing is back to normal.

"Did you eat today?" I ask.

He shakes his head.

He doesn't want to go to the hospital so we sit there with him while his wife makes him some pasta and sets it in front of him and he starts to eat. We have her make an appointment with his doctor for the next day and promise to see that he eats and checks his sugar regularly. They both thank us.

"I never get tired of seeing dextrose work," Arthur says. "It makes me feel like we're making a difference."

"I hear you," I say.


We're sent to a nursing home for a man just diagnosed with tuberculosis. We have to wear personal protective gear, OSHA-approved HEPA masks that make us look like characters from some science fiction movie. We breathe in and out like Darth Vader and the mask sucks in and out. We stand over the man who is looking at us like we are crazy. "We have come to take you from this sector," I say, in a fake computer-modulated voice. "Watches synchronized. Time is of the essence."

The man laughs.

"Resistance is futile," Arthur says. "Surrender to the dark side."

The man is laughing hysterically as we wheel him into the elevator, keeping our dialogue running.

A maintenance man steps in, sees our masks, then steps out quickly.

"We'll have to come back and kill him," I say.

Arthur pushes the button for the ground floor. "Escape hatch deployed."


In the afternoon, we are sent to pick up a woman with Alzheimer's at another nursing home. She has fallen and broken

**280**    **Peter Canning**

her hip. "This could be our last nursing-home tour together," I say, "Except when I visit you in a few years."

"Let's get them stirred up."

We do the routine up and down the halls with excellent response, lots of smiles and hellos. Coming back with the patient, just as we hit the exit, a short old man looks up and says, "Who you got there?"

"We're coming back for you," Arthur says.

"Fuck you, you are, fuck you in spades," he says.

"Well, isn't that nice."

"Up your kiester for Easter."

"What a pleasure meeting you, sir," Arthur says.

"Not for me," he says, "not for me at all."

"Losing your touch," I say.

Arthur shakes his head. "You gotta love these places."

At the end of the day, we finish up our paperwork, then meet at the time clock. "Well, Pedro," he says, "it's been fun."

"I swear I won't miss you," I say.

He offers his hand and a broad smile. We shake warmly.

"Have a good weekend," he says.

"You, too, old man," I say. "My friend."

I'm driving home up I-91 when a car comes up fast behind me, flashes me. I look to the side and see Arthur pull into the next lane. He smiles, gives me a salute, then roars on ahead.


# Life


It's night. A full moon is visible at the end of Albany Avenue, lit up all yellow and orange. Like outer space sitting on the city's shoulder. It's one of those moments that make me stop and appreciate what I am doing. Life here on Earth.

\* \* \*

The call is for a baby who choked but is now breathing. On the third floor of a tenement we find a father holding the child, a baby of just seven days, in a pink blanket. It is the middle of the night. He says she vomited up her milk and had trouble breathing. The baby is on AZT, an anti-AIDS medication. The baby is so tiny, I do not want to say everything is okay. I am not a father, although I share this new father's fear and concern. I listen to the baby's lungs, which are clear. I listen to her tiny heartbeat. I look into her eyes, which are barely open. "What hospital?" I say.

"Saint Francis."

I hold the baby in her blanket as the father gets in the ambulance, then I pass her up to my partner, who secures her on the stretcher in case we have a wreck, even though at this hour my headlights are the only ones on the night city streets.

Later I stand outside in the darkness and look in through the window of the ER waiting room. I see the father, rocking the baby slowly, whispering words I can't hear, sitting alone in a row of seats.

# The Job

Hartford has launched a project to knock down all of the estimated eight hundred abandoned buildings in the city limits. They've closed down two of the worst public housing complexes and are working on fixing up the third. Hartford, for all its problems, is a good city, one that I care about. There are good people here. I think about Mrs. Mays, her family, and the neighborhood deacon. She passed away in a convalescent home a few months after we took her to the hospital. As Arthur said when he read of her death, she is now undoubtedly dressed in her Sunday best, listening to harp music and walking in the garden with her Lord.

I get called for a woman with a sprained ankle and find it is the snake girl, who is now seven months pregnant. I ask her about the bunny in the cage; she says the snake got out and ate him. Does she still want a monkey? I ask.

She nods. "I know a place in Philly they will sell me one, but I want to have the baby first, and let him get grown a little before I bring a monkey in the house."

I am responding to a woman not feeling well, and when I notice her husband, a legless man in a wheelchair, I say, "Hey didn't you used to live over on Hudson Street?"

"Yeah, yeah," he says.

"You're Joe, right?"

"Yeah, yeah, that's me."

"How's the heart?"

"The old ticker's beating strong," he says.

He is concerned about his wife, who has been growing weak lately. We put her on the stretcher and he wheels up beside her, puts his arms around her, gives her a big kiss that causes her to blush. "These boys'll take good care of you, honey. Ain't that right, boys?"

Rebecca gets her second code save. Pam Duguay becomes a medic, and I get called to back her up on her first code. She gets the tube, and an EJ, and we run through the drug box trying to revive the woman. Then Matt Lincoln and I do a power lift, rapidly carrying the large woman down three flights of narrow stairs without stopping. At the hospital, the doctor compliments Pam on a good effort. She beams and gives me a hug in the hallway, thanking me for helping. I am in the middle of the company in terms of experience now. I think of those with more years than me—Daniel Tauber, Meg and Rick Domina, Rick Ortyl—and of how they have helped me and others, spreading the craft, passing it on. I think about all the newer medics—Rebecca, Todd Beaton, Matt Hannon, Chaz Milner—and watch them gaining confidence, saving lives.

There are days when I wonder about my future, what I am doing with myself and my life. I keep asking myself—shouldn't I be in some other line of work? Something safer, more secure, with stability. But I ignore those worries and they pass, at least for a while longer.

I stay working nights. I like watching the sun go down, then responding through the night, red lights whirling through the dark streets, answering calls for help. Just off Albany Avenue Chaz Milner and Missy Young deliver their second baby in two weeks. Annette O'Callaghan and Chris Bates respond to a chest pain on Park Terrace. On Squire Street Joe Stefano and Matt Rynaski work a shooting. Up on Tower, John Burelle and Jennifer Sabatini treat a young girl with asthma. Mark Bassett, Mike Carl, and Kim Quinn clear from their calls and go back on line. Downtown Chris Dennis loads a man with critical stab wounds into his ambulance and treats him while his partner, Dawn Jewiss, drives lights and sirens to the trauma center.

I sit in a parking lot overlooking the highway and the capitol, and watch the Life Star helicopter rise over the city skyline, its bright lights shining, heading out to the countryside where a volunteer ambulance crew is treating a patient trapped in a car.

Catherine Getlein, our dispatcher, calls my number, and my new partner, Kristin Shea, hits the lights on and we're off on a priority one—difficulty breathing.

We are in a tenement. I touch the man's forehead, which is hot and moist. I listen to his lungs, which are decreased in sound. I talk to him in Spanish. His wife looks at me and says, "You like your job, don't you?"

I am a little taken aback by her English and her words. "Yes," I say, "I do. *Me gusta mi trabajo.*"

She smiles. "I can tell," she says.

We give him oxygen and carry him down the stairs, and though my back is tired, I stand a little bit taller on this night. "They'll take good care of you here," I tell him at the hospital, touching his shoulder with my hand.

"Thank you," he says.

I head back out into the night.

# Postscript

Public Health Commissioner Stephen Harriman withdrew his name for renomination to a second term as head of the department hours after an explosive public hearing in which legislators castigated him for his poor oversight of emergency medical services systems in the state.

After an exposé in the *Hartford Courant*, the city paid for medical dispatch training for all its EMS dispatchers. Understaffing remains troublesome.

Our union membership approved a four-year contract with our new company after voting down the first two contract offers. While the new contract limits raises for paramedics to 3 percent, it maintains full health benefits for all employees who have worked full-time for four years.

# Acknowledgments

I would like to thank the men and women I work with on the road for their friendship and commitment to patient care. They remain the heart of the EMS system and anyone interested in improving the EMS system should listen to their voices and experience. This includes our company dispatchers.

Thank you to my medical control at Saint Francis Hospital, Dr. Michael Gutman. Also thanks to Hartford Hospital Medical Control, Dr. Sara Knuth, and other physicians who take the time to help paramedics. We appreciate the broadness of the paramedic guidelines sponsored jointly by the two hospitals.

Thank you to all the ER nurses at Saint Francis, Hartford Hospital, Mount Sinai, and Connecticut Children's Medical Center, who are overworked and probably underpaid, but who still seem to always manage smiles for their patients and for us. Thanks also to the clerical personnel and ER technicians.

Thank you to the dispatchers, Hartford police officers, and firefighters who assist us.

Thank you to Angela Griffin and the Lives-At-Risk project at Saint Francis and Jackie Grogan and the Children's ER, passionate advocates for their worthy programs.

Thank you to my friends, Barbara Danley, Ross Wheeler, and Kristin Oberg for reading and commenting on the manuscript. Their insights and support are invaluable.

Thanks to my agent, Jane Dystel and my editor, Susan Randol.

And most of all, thanks to Michelle.

*Read Peter Canning's first book . . .*

# PARAMEDIC
## On the Front Lines of Medicine

"Absorbing."
—*Publishers Weekly*

In this unforgettable, dramatic account of one man's experience as an EMT, Peter Canning relives the nerve-racking seconds that can mean the difference between a patient's death and survival, as Canning struggles to make the right call, dispense the right medication, or keep a patient's heart beating long enough to reach the hospital. As Canning tells his graphic, gripping war stories—of the lives he saved and lost; of the fear, the nightmares, and the constant adrenaline-pumping thrill of action—we come away with an unforgettable portrait of what it means to be a hero.

Published by The Random House Publishing Group.
Available in bookstores everywhere.

# EMT
## Beyond the Lights and Sirens

## by Pat Foley

*Experience the rush of adrenaline
and the pain of loss.*

Pat Foley takes you inside the ambulance and on
the road with volunteer rescue personnel. Witness
the courage and compassion that makes the EMT
an unsung hero in some of the most vital and com-
pelling medical dramas of our time.

# TRAUMA CENTER

## by Joan E. Lloyd
## & Edwin B. Herman

*The front lines of emergency medicine—
from the EMT units to the ER*

Emergency Medical Response Teams. Whether in
the air, on the road, or in the ER, every day they
face split-second decisions—and one false move
can mean the difference between life and death.